PALLIATIVE CARE FOR CHILDREN AND FAMILIES

Palliative Care for Children and Families

An Interdisciplinary Approach

Edited by

Jayne Price and Patricia McNeilly

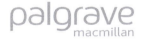

First published 2009 by
PALGRAVE MACMILLAN

Palgrave Macmillan in the UK is an imprint of Macmillan Publishers Limited, registered in England, company number 785998, of Houndmills, Basingstoke, Hampshire RG21 6XS.

Palgrave Macmillan in the US is a division of St Martin's Press LLC, 175 Fifth Avenue, New York, NY 10010.

Palgrave Macmillan is the global academic imprint of the above companies and has companies and representatives throughout the world.

Palgrave and Macmillan are registered trademarks in the United States, the United Kingdom, Europe and other countries

ISBN 978–0–230–20002–9

This book is printed on paper suitable for recycling and made from fully managed and sustained forest sources. Logging, pulping and manufacturing processes are expected to conform to the environmental regulations of the country of origin.

A catalogue record for this book is available from the British Library.

10   9   8   7   6   5   4   3   2   1
18   17   16   15   14   13   12   11   10   09

Printed and bound in Great Britain by CPI Antony Rowe, Chippenham and Eastbourne

2/9/10

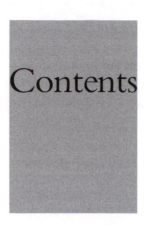

Contents

Foreword by Sir Alan Craft   vii

Preface   ix

Acknowledgements   xi

Notes on the Contributors   xiv

Chapter 1   **Palliative Care for Children a Unique Way of Caring**   1
                Jayne Price and Marisa McFarlane

Chapter 2   **Interdisciplinary Working**   18
                Patricia McNeilly and Frances Gilmore

Chapter 3   **Communicating Effectively**   38
                Jayne Price and Carole Cairns

Chapter 4   **Ethical Issues**   64
                Helen E. Bennett

Chapter 5   **Meeting the Spiritual Needs of Children and Families**   88
                Wilfred McSherry and Sue Jolley

Chapter 6   **Supporting Children and Families**   107
                Fiona Collinson and Karen Bleakley

Chapter 7   **Reflection – Advancing Care and Practice**   128
                Patricia McNeilly and Jayne Price

Chapter 8   **Symptom Management**   142
                Heather McCluggage and Satbir Singh Jassal

Chapter 9   **Care of the Child at the End of Life**   172
Ruth Davies

Chapter 10   **Bereavement Care**   192
Jenni Thomas OBE and Ann Chalmers

Chapter 11   **Future Directions for Children's Palliative Care**   213
Sharon McCloskey and Lizzie Chambers

Index   229

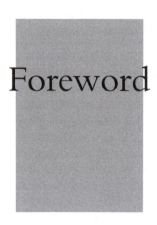

Foreword

Palliative care for children is a relatively new concept and in many ways is very different from adult palliative care. Palliative care for children grew out of the need to provide good symptom care for children with cancer, but has developed to be very much more than that. It is a speciality in its own right, but is also becoming an integral part of the care of children and young people with many chronic conditions.

The ACT definition of children's palliative care is:

> An active and total approach to care, embracing physical, emotional, social and spiritual elements. It focuses on enhancement of quality of life for the child and support for the family and includes management of distressing symptoms, provision of respite and care through death and bereavement.

This, of course, also applies to young people as well as children. Palliative care is not just something that comes in at the end of life, but is a thread that runs through the lives of children with many chronic illnesses and disabilities.

The group of children and young people who need such services are mainly those who have life-threatening or life-limiting conditions. While attempts have been made to define these situations, they are not perfect, and a definition based on need is probably just as valid:

> Life-limiting conditions are those for which there is no reasonable hope of cure and from which children or young people will die. Some of these conditions cause progressive deterioration, rendering the child increasingly dependent on parents and carers.
>
> Life-threatening conditions are those for which curative treatment may be feasible but can fail, such as cancer. Children in long term remission or following successful curative treatment are not included.

Palliative care is not the province of one group of practitioners, and the basics are something that needs to be grasped by all professions caring for children. I am pleased to see this new book, which recognizes the need to broaden the scope of children's palliative care and covers the many facets of the subject.

There are many professionals who come into contact with a child and his or her family where there is a life-threatening or life-limiting condition. All are experts in their own field but all are also interdependent on the work of other practitioners. Palliative care is a daunting subject for many, can cause real anxiety and distress in the practitioner and this can be transmitted to the child and family. A better knowledge of palliative care for all will empower professionals to cope with their own input into the child's care, and to better interact with the myriads of others involved in any particular situation. What parents want are professionals who are knowledgeable, competent and confident in what they are doing. They also do not want to have to explain again to the next professional who comes along what has gone before.

This book is an important contribution to the growing educational material that is available, both for those who wish to specialize in palliative care and for all of those who are involved in any way with these children, young people and their families.

Palliative care in children is not just about dying. It is about the need to make the best of living whatever may be round the corner, and however long or short that life might be.

The pioneer of adult palliative care, Cicely Saunders, said:

How people die lives on in the memories of those left behind.

What we must all strive for is to ensure the best possible memories of life and as comfortable a death as is possible.

This book will help us all to achieve that aim.

SIR ALAN CRAFT
Professor of Child Health
University of Newcastle upon Tyne

This Foreword is an edited extract from Craft, A. W. and Killen, S. (2007) *Palliative Care Services for Children and Young People in England*, Department of Health, May.

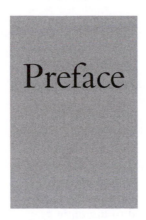

Preface

The provision of palliative care for children and their families has gained momentum in recent years, both within the United Kingdom and further afield. This has been reflected by the increasing number of services and individuals within those services, both statutory and voluntary, who have worked tirelessly to improve and develop care in this field of practice, in partnership with those who use them. The need for professionals and others to work in a collaborative way around the needs of children and families has never been greater, hence the emphasis on interdisciplinary working throughout the course of this text.

In this book we have brought together the expertise of a wide variety of practitioners, academics and researchers from across the UK, who have drawn on their knowledge and experience to highlight the crucial issues that come to the fore when caring for children who are life-limited, life-threatened or in the end stages of life. In doing so, the perspective of the parent has also been included; in Chapter 9, Ruth Davies discusses the care of the child who is dying, from her own perspective as a parent, in addition to her experience as a children's nurse and as a researcher. Indeed, she has dedicated this chapter to the memory of her beloved son, Tomos, 17.4.1987–3.08.2006.

Alongside the increase of service provision for children with palliative care needs and their families, has been the much needed increase in the research base underpinning practice within the field in recent years. While further research is ongoing and future work planned, this text draws together much of the research evidence currently available from a national and international perspective on which to guide and base practice.

This text is designed to assist all those who work with children who have palliative care needs and their families, on a regular or an occasional basis. This will include students undertaking both undergraduate and postgraduate education programmes within health and social care, in addition to those already working in this area of practice. While the editors acknowledge that, given the large number of individuals who make up the interdisciplinary team, it would be impossible to include the role of every person who might be involved in children's palliative care, it is anticipated that most feature at some point within the text.

Because the many authors who contributed to this book come from varied backgrounds, it is not surprising, given the holistic nature of the subject area, that at times there is some overlap between chapters, though often this highlights differing perspectives. Each chapter includes a number of engaging features; for example, readers may be directed towards further reading, or asked to undertake an activity requiring them to reflect on their own practice or experiences. Similarly, readers are at times directed to relevant web pages for further information. Key points are also used to highlight relevant issues, and a summary box is included at the end of each chapter to tie together the main messages. Also included are clinical scenarios detailing the care of a child and family, some of which feature the role of a particular individual, for example the Paediatrician, Community Children's Nurse or Funeral Director, while others incorporate the roles of numerous individuals. It should be stressed from the outset that these scenarios are fictitious, and have been used to discuss issues that may arise in the course of caring for such children; any similarities to real-life situations have occurred by chance. Although readers may wish to read the book from cover to cover, it is equally useful to study or refer to individual chapters as the need arises. It is acknowledged that those working in this field may be involved with very young children, or with those having reached adolescence; however, the term 'children' is used throughout this text to refer to both children and young people. 'Interdisciplinary' is used as a term that includes voluntary or other agencies as well as professionals.

The editors are indebted to all those who have contributed to this book, for their enthusiasm, patience, dedication and reliability. We would also like to thank Lynda Thompson and Kate Llewellyn (Palgrave Macmillan) for their support throughout this process, and Paddy Haughian (Queen's University Belfast) for his input in the final stages of the book.

The impetus for editing this book was to provide a useful addition to the small number of texts about children's palliative care, and to enhance the current thinking of professionals working across the interdisciplinary interface. We hope this book will become a key resource for all those working with children who have palliative care needs, in partnership with their families, to assist them to meet challenges, with the ultimate aim of enhancing the quality of care.

JAYNE PRICE
PATRICIA McNEILLY

Acknowledgements

The authors, editors and publishers wish to thank the following for permission to reproduce copyright material:

Chapter 1

Lizzie Chambers (ACT), for Figure 1.2: Principles of children's palliative care, from ACT (Association of Children with Life-threatening or Terminal Conditions and their Families) (2004) *A Framework for the Development of Integrated Multi-Agency Care Pathways for Children with Life-Threatening and Life-limiting Conditions.* Bristol: ACT.

International Journal of Palliative Nursing, for Figure 1.3: The uniqueness of children's palliative care, from J. Price, P. McNeilly, and M. McFarlane (2005) Paediatric palliative care in the UK: past, present and future. *International Journal of Palliative Nursing*, **11**(3): 124–9.

Chapter 2

European Journal of Palliative Care for Figure 2.3: An example of the children's palliative care team, from P. McNeilly and J. Price (2007) Interdisciplinary team-working in paediatric palliative care, *European Journal of Palliative Care*, **14**(2): 64–7.

Lizzie Chambers, ACT, for Figure 2.6: Standards: ICP for children with life-threatening and life-limiting conditions, from Association of Children with Life-limiting, Life-threatening and Terminal Conditions and their Families (2004) *A Framework for the Development of Integrated Multi-agency Care Pathways for Children with Life-threatening and Life-limiting Conditions,* Bristol: ACT.

Chapter 3

Cancer Nursing Practice, for Figure 3.5: The specific information needs of children, from J. Price (2003) Information needs of the child with cancer and their family, *Cancer Nursing Practice*, **2**(7): 35–8.

Chapter 4

Royal College of Paediatrics and Child Health, for Figure 4.4: Five situations . . . , from RCPCH (2004) *Withholding or Withdrawing Life Sustaining Treatment in Children. A Framework for Practice*, 2nd edn. London: RCPCH.

Chapter 5

Oxford University Press, for Table 5.1: Distinguishing the concepts of religion and spirituality, from H. G. Koenig, M. E. McCullough and D. B. Larson (2001) *Handbook of Religion and Health*, Oxford University Press.

Jessica Kingsley Publishers Ltd, for Figure 5.1: Spirituality as a football, from W. McSherry (2006) *Making Sense of Spirituality in Nursing and Health Care Practice: An Interactive Approach*.

Jessica Kingsley Publishers Ltd, for Table 5.2: Children's spiritual needs, adapted from W. McSherry (2006) *Making Sense of Spirituality in Nursing and Health Care Practice: An Interactive Approach*, pp. 567.

Paediatric Nursing/RCN Publishing Company, for Table 5.3: Children's expressions of spiritual needs, adapted from W. McSherry and J. Smith (2007) How do children express their spiritual needs?, *Paediatric Nursing*, **19**(3): 17–20.

Chapter 6

The Stationery Office for Figure 6.2: Framework for assessment of children in need and their families, reproduced with the permission of the Controller of HMSO and Queen's Printer for Scotland.

Chapter 7

This chapter is reproduced from P. McNeilly, J. Price and S. McCloskey (2006) A model for reflection in children's palliative care, *European Journal of Palliative Care*, **13**(1): 31–4, with kind permission.

Chapter 8

Jassal, S. (2008) *Basic Symptom Control in Paediatric Palliative Care: The Rainbows Hospice Guidelines* (7th edn), available from www.act.org.uk. The material reproduced in this chapter is by Satbir Singh Jassal and is reproduced with his permission.

World Health Organization, for Figure 8.4: WHO pain ladder, WHO, *Cancer Pain Relief and Palliative Care in Children* (1998).

Chapter 9

Lizzie Chambers (ACT), for Figure 9.1: End-of-life care pathway, from Association for Children with Life-threatening or Terminal Conditions and their Families (2004) *A Framework for the Development of Integrated Multi-agency Care Pathways for Children with Life-threatening and Life-limiting Conditions,* Bristol, ACT.

Chapter 10

Child Bereavement Charity, for Clinical Focus, excerpt from A. Chalmers (ed.) (2008) *Farewell, My Child*, Child Bereavement Charity, West Wycombe.

Anne Chalmers, CEO, Child Bereavement Charity, for Figure 10.1: Chinese pictogram for listening.

Professor M. Stroebe, for Figure 10.2: A dual process model for coping with bereavement.

Chapter 11

Lizzie Chambers, (ACT) for Figure 11.2: Three stages of an integrated multi-agency care pathway.

Figure 11.3: The Leaving Cone Model, reproduced with the kind permission of the ACT and Children's Hospices UK Education and Training Working Party, and Dr Linda Maynard, Head of Education and Development, East Anglia's Children's Hospices.

Every effort has been made to contact all copyright-holders, but if any have been inadvertently omitted the publishers will be pleased to make the necessary arrangement at the earliest opportunity.

Notes on the Contributors

Helen Bennett, Care Manager, Naomi House Children's Hospice, UK.

Karen Bleakley, Palliative Care Nurse Specialist (Paediatric), Paediatric Palliative Nurse Lecturer, Practice Educator, Northern Ireland Hospice Care.

Dr Carole Cairns, Staff Grade in Paediatric Haematology/Oncology, Royal Belfast Hospital for Sick Children.

Ann Chalmers, Chief Executive, Child Bereavement Charity.

Lizzie Chambers, Chief Executive, ACT (Association for Children's Palliative Care).

Fiona Collinson, Social Worker, Royal Belfast Hospital for Sick Children.

Dr Ruth Davies, Senior Lecturer (Nursing), Swansea University, Wales.

Frances Gilmore, Lead Nurse for Children's Services, Western Health and Social Care Trust, Northern Ireland.

Dr Satbir Singh Jassal, Medical Director, Rainbows Children's Hospice, and General Practitioner.

Sue Jolley, Lecturer in Paediatric Nursing, University of Hull.

Sharon McCloskey, Care Team Manager, Northern Ireland Hospice Care.

Dr Heather McCluggage, Associate Specialist in Paediatric Palliative Care, Western Health and Social Care Trust, Northern Ireland.

Marisa McFarlane, Paediatric Macmillan Nurse, Belfast Health and Social Care Trust.

Patricia McNeilly, Teaching Fellow, School of Nursing and Midwifery, Queen's University of Belfast.

Professor Wilfred McSherry, Faculty of Health, Staffordshire University.

Jayne Price, Sandra Ryan Research Fellow/ Senior Teaching Fellow, School of Nursing and Midwifery, Queen's University of Belfast.

Jenni Thomas OBE, Founder and President, Child Bereavement Charity.

The editors would also like to recognize contributions from:

Jill Clarke, Children's Occupational Therapist, Northern Health and Social Care Trust, Northern Ireland.

Elizabeth Gillespie, Community Children's Nurse Team Leader, Children's and Young People's Specialist Services, East Community Health Partnership Glasgow, Scotland.

Peter C. Mulholland, Funeral Home Manager, Mulhollands of Carrickfergus, Northern Ireland.

Sophie Rea, Hospital Play Specialist, Children's Haematology Unit , Royal Belfast Hospital for Sick Children, Northern Ireland.

Ursula Sheerin, Speech and Language Therapist, Northern Ireland.

Naomi Spence, CLIC Sargent Community Play Specialist, Belfast Northern Ireland.

Palliative Care for Children – a Unique Way of Caring

Jayne Price and Marisa McFarlane

Introduction

Palliative care for children is an integrated approach to care which ensures quality of life for children for whom an early death is expected (Liben *et al.* 2008). This philosophy of care is premised on a quality of living for both the child whose life is limited and for their family (ACT 2003). The central aim is to achieve quality for the duration of the individual child's life and a dignified death for the child in a place that is preferably the choice of the child and family (ACT 2007a).

In recent years, children's palliative care has emerged as a small but distinct area of practice from a national and global perspective (ACT 1997, Hutchinson *et al.* 2003, ACT 2003, Hynson *et al.* 2003, Sourkes *et al.* 2005). This development has not been without challenges, however, because of the different needs of children and families; the variation in availability of services depending on geographical location; a lack of understanding by policy-makers about what constitutes palliative care; difficulty in recognizing which children require this approach to care, and the small but increasing numbers of these children.

Palliative care for children has its roots in the hospice movement, and this flexible approach to care is now delivered in a variety of settings – at home, in hospital or in hospices. Huge progress has undoubtedly been made in the past twenty-five years, and the recent independent review (Craft and Killen 2007) endorses this. The number of professionals with an interest in palliative care for children has increased alongside a more established interdisciplinary and interagency network (Hain and Wallace 2008). Collaborative working and strategic policy development has been crucial. However, the need for continued developments for these children and families has been reinforced, and the future requirement for service provision has never been clearer. Key policy and strategic documents outline the commitment to improving care and services for these children and families in the future (IOM 2002, ACT 2003, DH 2005, Craft and Killen 2007, DHSSPS 2007, DH 2008).

This opening chapter sets the scene for the book by tracing the development of the field of practice known as children's palliative care from a historical perspective, and investigates which children require a palliative approach to care. We also examine the legislation underpinning and guiding the continuous development of this speciality, and unravel the philosophy of caring while setting it in context of the very unique and challenging needs of both children and families.

KEY POINT

Recognition of the unique needs of children requiring palliative care has increased nationally and internationally in recent years.

Children's palliative care – definitions and categories

An independent review of palliative care services for children and young people in England, carried out for the Secretary of State (Craft and Killen 2007), reinforced the belief that there was a lack of understanding of what children's palliative care involved, with many assuming it was exclusively about end-of-life care. McCulloch *et al.* (2008) further endorsed this, emphasizing that palliative care for children is not simply provision at the end of their lives, but is rather a continuum of care, including responsive services and specialist services.

The word 'palliate' has its etymological root in Latin, being derived from the word 'pallium', which means a cloak or shroud. 'Pallium' was moderated to become 'palliate', which means 'to cloak, shelter or clothe'. The notion of providing a cloak or a shelter, is therefore particularly appropriate for a family systems approach to the care of a child nearing the end of life and their family, with the family surrounding and cloaking the ill child (Rallison and Moules 2004).

While a variety of definitions exist, one that is commonly used is by the Association for Children with Life-Threatening or Terminal Conditions and their Families, (renamed in 2004 as the Association for Children's Palliative Care) (ACT) and Royal College of Paediatrics and Child Health (RCPCH). It summarizes children's palliative care as:

> An active and total approach to care, embracing physical, emotional, social and spiritual elements. It focuses on enhancement of quality life for the child and support for the family and includes the management of distressing symptoms, provision of respite and care through death and bereavement (ACT and RCPCH 2003: 9).

Palliative care for children is therefore a multidimensional approach consisting of many aspects of care in addition to end-of-life care, which may be delivered for the duration of the child's life and for years beyond. In this definition, quality of life is the prime concern, not death.

As the speciality continues to develop, so does the debate, confusion and ambiguity about the terms used within children's palliative care. Rallison *et al.* (2006) challenge the commonly used terms of 'life-limiting' and 'life-threatening', suggesting that these terms emphasize a threat and a limitation may not in fact capture the children's and families' whole experience. In addition, they encourage consideration that the use of this language may be dangerous as it sets this group of children apart from others having a life defined by illness. The terms 'hospice care' and 'palliative care' are often used interchangeably (Steele *et al.* 2008). In an attempt to differentiate the terms and provide clarity, Lamers (2002) asserts that all hospice care is palliative care, but all palliative care is not hospice care. Palliative care is therefore seen as a broad philosophy of care, whereas hospice care is a specific model for delivering palliative care. The fact that terms within this area of practice are used interchangeably was reported by Nicholl (2007) in a study interviewing nurses working with these children and their families. These terms included: complex needs, life-limiting, life-threatening, palliative care and so on, and confusion prevails despite the existence of common definitions as offered by ACT and RCPCH (1997, 2003).

It has been recognized that palliative care for children is provided to children with life-limiting conditions for whom curative treatment is not available or no longer appropriate (ACT and RCPCH 2003). Life-limiting conditions can be described as:

> conditions for which there is no reasonable hope of cure and from which children or young people will die (ACT and RCPCH 1997, 2003: 9).

Many of the life-limiting conditions are characterized by progressive deterioration, which in turns requires more intensive care from parents and carers. A life-threatening condition can be described as:

> an illness for which curative treatment may be feasible but can fail (ACT and RCPCH 2003: 9).

Children requiring a palliative approach to care have been classified as delineating into four broad groups (see Figure 1.1) (ACT and RCPCH 1997, 2003). This has been vital in the development and provision of services since the inception of the classifications in 1997. The classifications are internationally accepted and help us to see the types of conditions that mean a child needs palliative care. The classification outlines the expected trajectory within each group rather than providing a complete list of all life-limiting conditions (Hain and Wallace 2008).

The illness trajectory for a child with a life-threatening illness such as cancer (Group 1) and their family can be characterized by periods of hope, where treatment is successful for some time, after which a relapse may occur, then further treatment options may generate new hope for the child and family. A life-threatening illness may indeed become life-limiting when all treatment options have been exhausted.

Children with a diagnosis falling into Groups 2, 3 or 4 have an illness where no treatment is available, where life is limited and death is normally inevitable in childhood.

> *Group 1* Life-threatening conditions for which curative treatment may be feasible but can fail. Palliative care may be necessary during periods of prognostic uncertainty and when treatment fails: for example, cancer, irreversible organ failures of heart, liver, kidney.
>
> *Group 2* Conditions where there may be long periods of intensive treatment aimed at prolonging life and allowing participation in normal childhood activities, but premature death is still possible: for example, cystic fibrosis, muscular dystrophy.
>
> *Group 3* Progressive conditions without curative treatment options, where treatment is exclusively palliative and may commonly extend over many years: for example, Batten's disease, mucopolysaccharidosis.
>
> *Group 4* Conditions with severe neurological disability which may cause weakness and susceptibility to health complications, and may deteriorate unpredictably, but are not considered progressive: for example, multiple disabilities, such as brain or spinal cord injuries, including severe cerebral palsy.

Figure 1.1   Classifications of children requiring palliative care
Source: ACT and RCPCH (1997, 2003).

Liben *et al.* (2008) identify that despite a number of definitions of children's palliative care being published, the remaining challenge is to create a definition which straddles the boundaries of all cultures and nations.

═══ WEB LINK ═══

Access the International Children's Palliative Care Network's website at www.icpcn. org.uk to identify the current position regarding the key definitions used within children's palliative care.

The prevalence of children requiring palliative care

Given the broad diagnostic mix of children with palliative care needs, it is very difficult to obtain a full picture of the exact numbers of such children. Registers in existence give statistics for specific illnesses – for example, cancer and cerebral palsy registers – but many of the rarer life-limiting conditions may not be recorded anywhere. While figures are important in assessing need and planning future service development, the fact that these children have not previously been considered as a specific group, and therefore a separate data base relating to them does not exist, further complicates the situation (Hutchinson *et al.* 2003). Estimates from the United Kingdom (UK) in 2003 suggested that at least twelve children in every 10,000 have a life-limiting condition and will die before adulthood (ACT 2003). Furthermore, the estimates also indicate that these figures are set to increase in future years (ACT and RCPCH 2003). Recent estimates for England indicate a prevalence rate of sixteen per 10,000 if neonatal conditions are included, and fifteen per 10,000 if they are excluded (Craft and Killen 2007). For the UK as a whole, Children's Hospices UK predict that 20,000–25,000 families are living with the reality that their child is going to die before adulthood (Children's Hospices UK 2008). Worldwide, it is estimated that at least seven million children could benefit from palliative care, but access to such services remains inconsistent across countries for both children and their families (ICPCN 2007).

The development of children's palliative care could be attributed to increasing demand, brought about partly by the improved survival rate of children with complex health needs (Hewitt-Taylor 2005). This is a group of children who would previously have died early (Steele 2000) but who now survive longer, often as a result of advances in medical interventions and new technologies. Despite this, however, many of these children still have a limited life span. It is clear that there is an overlap with children who have a disability, those who have complex needs and those who require palliative care. The Department of Health (Craft and Killen 2007) suggests that palliative care for children should be considered as a strand that runs through the lives of many children who have disabilities and complex needs. Some children who have a disability or complex problems will not be life-limited, while others will be.

Another group of children who require palliative care are those with advanced malignant disease. The prognosis for children with cancer has improved greatly over recent years. Medical advances have had a part to play in improved survival rates, particularly complex drug protocols and combinations of different treatment modalities. Despite these advances in the treatment of childhood cancers, however, approximately 30 per cent of children suffering from cancer in the United Kingdom still die as a result of their illness and will require a purely palliative approach to care (Vickers *et al.* 2007).

Today in developed countries, death in childhood is a relatively rare occurrence (Goldman 2007), which may also in part be a result of the reduction of acute diseases through vaccinations, improved housing and better standards of living. It is precisely this lack of frequency and raised expectations for health and well-being that can make it even more difficult for families, health care professionals and the wider community to accept the death of a child (Hynson *et al.* 2003).

While the numbers of children requiring palliative care is a relatively small, this group of children and their families require intense and sustained support and specialist services, not only for the duration of the child's life, but also for several years beyond.

Historical development

Children's palliative care has developed from the hospice movement and now sits as a small but distinct area of practice in its own right. By the early 1980s there were over sixty adult hospice-type services in the UK, and the hospice approach was inspirational in the provision of end-of-life care. However, the need for further service expansion was soon identified, from simply providing care for adult cancer patients to addressing the needs of children and young people. The growth of child-specific services soon followed, including the further development of outreach teams from children's oncology units and the opening of the world's first children's hospice. The need for a hospice specifically for children grew from a special bond of friendship between Sister Frances Dominica and a child called Helen, who had a life-limiting illness. Sister Frances Dominica's vision was for a haven where both the practical support so needed by families and respite care could be delivered within the ethos of family-centred care. In 1982, the first children's hospice, Helen House, was opened in Oxford, to provide a 'home for home' where families could share the caring in an environment where practical help, friendship and quality time were offered. This was to 'blaze a trail in the provision of hospice care for children and young people' (Worswick 2000: 160) in the UK, and world wide since that time. Helen House has served as an exemplar for the development of most of the subsequent children's hospices that have been opened (Lenton *et al.* 2006). A steady growth in the number of children's hospices in the UK followed, as well as the development of 'hospice at home' teams, which added to established home care already provided for children with cancer (Lauer and Camitta 1980, Goldman *et al.* 1990).

In 1992, ACT (the Association for Children with Life-Threatening or Terminal Conditions and their Families, since renamed the Association for Children's Palliative Care) was set up, to influence and promote excellence and equality in care provision and support for children and young people with life-threatening or life-limiting conditions and their families. As a national charity, ACT looks to achieve its aims through campaigning for improved provision of palliative care services for children and families, and working with professionals to support the delivery of the best care possible while empowering families to make their voices heard in the development of future services.

Alongside these developmentss there was increased interest from professionals regarding the specific needs of children with life-limiting/life-threatening illnesses and their families.

WEB LINK

Go to www.act.org.uk and familiarize yourself with the work currently being carried out by ACT within the field of children's palliative care since its inception and more recently.

The charity works closely with other agencies and organizations, including the Association of Children's Hospices UK (previously the Association of Children's Hospices – ACH), which was established as an official charity in 1998.

In the intervening years since the inception of ACT, the organization, in collaboration with others (including other organizations, professionals and families), has made a significant impact on the understanding and acknowledgement of child and family needs, and on the improvement and development of care through publications, reports, guidelines for good practice, and care pathways. ACT in 1997 jointly with RCPCH published *A Guide to the Development of Children's Palliative Care Services* (ACT/RCPCH, 1997). This was a crucial document giving clear direction for future service development. Much work had been achieved by the 2nd edition of this document in 2003, although further scope for future improvements was outlined. At time of writing the 3rd edition is eagerly awaited further demonstrating how ACT continue to make a significant impact on the understanding and acknowledgement of need, and on the improvement and development of care.

The UK government too have shown their commitment to the continuing development of services for children requiring palliative care and their families has been outlined in the first ever strategy document, entitled' Better Care: Better Lives', which clearly maps the future direction of the speciality (DH 2008).

--- WEB LINK ---

Go to www.dh.gov.uk/en/Publicationsandstatistics/Publications/PublicationsPolicyAndGuidance/DH_083106 and familiarize yourself with the eight service development goals set out in 'Better Care: Better Lives'.

There is variability in care and services for children with palliative care needs worldwide, and Downing (2008) states the importance of considering models of care in low-resource areas under-developed countries. In recognition that children require high-quality palliative care services all over the world, ACT, in 2005, through international collaboration, set up the International Children's Palliative Care network Network (ICPCN). The aim of this network is to ensure that standards of palliative care for children are maintained across the global arena. In the spirit of the UN Convention (1989) decreeing that every child has the right to the highest standard of health, the ICPCN Charter (2008) has been devised and clearly sets out the international standard of support that is the right of all children living with life-limiting and life-threatening illnesses worldwide, and their families. It is hoped that ethos of this charter will be accepted and ratified by governments and health departments around the world, and reduce the inequity that currently exists.

--- WEB LINK ---

Go to www.act.org.uk/dmdocuments/ICPCN%20Charter.pdf to see the standards of support set out in the ICPCN Charter.

It is a commonly-held misconception that a hospice is a place for end-of-life care for children with cancer, but in fact children with malignancy and their families rarely use hospices (Vickers *et al.* 2007). However, the hospice remains an option for all children requiring palliative care, and provides all the dimensions of palliative care throughout the child's life, in addition to end-of-life care as necessary.

While palliative care for children has evolved from the hospice care philosophy, its focus now extends far beyond the care of the dying in a hospice setting (Himelstein *et al.* 2004) and palliative care for children is provided in hospitals, at home or in a hospice setting. It is seldom that a child will have their care provided in just one or other of these locations; moreover, many of these children may experience all three during the different stages of their palliative care journey.

================================ **ACTIVITY** ================================

Consider recent changes in the way palliative care has been delivered in your workplace/region.

The principles and philosophy of care

The philosophy of palliative care for children is thus premised on a holistic, individualized approach, centred around the unique needs of the individual child and
family during the child's limited life trajectory (Price *et al.* 2005). All children
requiring palliative care will have an individual care package which includes variable components of both generic and specialist palliative care provided in a
planned, co-ordinated, timely and flexible manner as needed (ICPCN 2007). It is
essential to recognize that care may be required over a protracted period, and be
delivered by a range of professionals straddling the interdisciplinary interface
(McNeilly and Price 2007), thus the need for a co-ordinated and structured
approach is paramount, with each member of team working towards a common
goal (see Chapter 2). The importance of a key worker has also been highlighted
(ACT 2003), as this professional can ensure the streamlining and cohesiveness of
the interdisciplinary approach to care. The principles of palliative care have been
suggested by ACT (2004) (see Figure 1.2).

When delivering palliative care to children, the family must be central. The
child with a life-limiting illness should be viewed within the context of

---

Principles of children's palliative care

■ Care should be child- and family-focused and should take into account the
child's rights.

■ Care should encompass symptom management, emotional support, practical support, spiritual needs and bereavement support for the whole family, and should
respect cultural and religious differences.

■ Service delivery should be based on assessment of needs, starting as soon as possible after diagnosis or recognition.

■ The delivery of care should be well co-ordinated, with an emphasis on continuity
of services.

■ Care plans should be flexible to accommodate changing needs and choices.

■ Regular review of needs should be undertaken, and care plans should be flexible to
accommodate changing needs and choices.

■ Regular reviews of needs should be undertaken, and care plans adjusted to take
into account changes in circumstances.

Figure 1.2 Principles of children's palliative care

Source: ACT (2004). Reproduced with the kind permission of ACT.

the family system and as such as a highly dependent entity within that family. The family is many things to the child, influencing his or her life, development and belief system. In addition, the family value system largely forms the child's meaning of life, illness and death (Bartell and Kissane 2005).

WEB LINK

Familiarize yourself with the documents produced by ACT and Children's Hospices UK to aid in the development of children's palliative care services, at: www.act.org.uk and www.childhospice.org.uk

---

Models of care

Provision of palliative care services for children and how they are delivered have developed greatly since the initial document *A Guide to the Development of Children's Palliative Care Services* (ACT 1997). While there has been an increase in home-based palliative care teams, children's hospices and strategic guidance in progressing this speciality (ACT 2003), there is still a large variation in the availability of these services, with access depending on local availability and funding (Craft and Killen 2007). One reason for this variability is that provision of palliative care for children and young people is provided by a network of agencies including the NHS, the voluntary sector, and the social and educational services (DH 2005).

In its review of services provided to children requiring palliative care and their families, ACT (2003) identified that the most established model of care was delivered to children with cancer. Paediatric oncology outreach nurse specialists (POONS) working from a tertiary or shared care centre are central to this approach to care. Their role is to provide a link between hospital and home, to promote a system of seamless care (Bignold *et al.* 1994). In palliative care, they offer advice on symptom management and support, not only to the child and family, but also to local community nurses and primary care teams. Medical support is provided by paediatric oncologists and haematologists, in collaboration with paediatricians, GPs, and adult or children's palliative care consultants (WMPMT 2005). In recent years, social workers, psychologists and play specialists based at regional hospitals have extended their services into the community (Price and Spence 2004).

The document entitled *Improving Outcomes in Children and Young People with Cancer* (NICE 2005) addresses some pertinent issues in relation to the palliative care needs of teenagers and young people. It recognizes that there are few dedicated services for this client group, that some community children's services do not accept referrals for patients aged over 16, and there is very limited hospice provision for young people. Indeed, this is true of respite care for young adults with non-malignant conditions, and is a major challenge, bringing with it issues such as transition to adult services. Indeed, Pfund (2007) concedes that achieving a workable model for this client group is still a long way off.

FURTHER READING

Read ACT (2007b) *The Transition Care Pathway: A Framework for the Development of Integrated Multi-Agency Care Pathways for Young People with Life-threatening and Life-limiting Conditions*, and consider the main principles outlined. Available at: www.act.org

Models of care offering community-based care for children and young people with palliative care needs are increasingly being established. This care is provided by teams involving, for example, paediatricians, occupational therapists, physiotherapists, dieticians, and speech and language therapists. Children's community nursing teams have been identified as being the bedrock of local service provision (Craft and Killen 2007, DH 2008), some of whom have a specialist remit for children's palliative care (Davies 1999). There is an emphasis on the need to ensure increased focus on community services 'to help manage and support children with palliative care needs to stay at home' (Craft and Killen 2007: 7). For this to occur, there need to be more flexible, comprehensive teams capable of providing care for twenty-four hours a day and seven days a week in the locality of the child and family.

Children's hospices provide flexible, family-centred care throughout a child's illness and after death. Hospice care is an approach to care rather than a place of care. It is founded on the belief that children and their families should be offered help to achieve a physical, emotional and spiritual quality of life (WMPMT 2005). Hospices vary in the services they provide and while mainly nurse-led, are interdisciplinary. They may provide planned or emergency respite, either in a hospice or at home, and palliative and bereavement support. Some may offer professional education. There are positive examples of hospices working in partnership with other agencies to improve and develop services available to children and their families, thus increasing choice in the preferred place of care (Farrell and Sutherland 1998, McCready Donnelly Lowry, 2007). While hospices receive very little statutory funding and rely on donations and grants, there is an increasing move to secure long-term funding (Children's Palliative Care Alliance 2008).

Finally, some reference has to be made to the number of children and young people with palliative care needs who die in hospital. The Department of Health (Craft and Killen 2007) indicates that in England the number of children dying in hospital is high (74 per cent), despite most families preferring the child's death to take place at home. Parents may lack choice because of restricted services and facilities. However, hospital may be the choice for those families needing a sense of security and support from a team with whom they are familiar (Goldman *et al.* 1990). There are instances where a child will forgo his or her preference when sensing the parents' inability to cope at home (Howell 1995).

In the past, curative and palliative approaches were viewed as being exclusive and independent entities; palliative care being considered as starting when curative treatment failed. This led to what Feudtner (2007) described as an abrupt transition from curative to palliative/supportive care; however, he also queried that a transition might never have been made. Early integration of palliative care seems crucial, and mixed management models of palliative care for children challenge service providers to offer a blended approach to care that includes a mix of disease-directed treatments and palliative care (Glare and Virik 2001, Hynson *et al.* 2003, Liben *et al.* 2008).

Current models of care are now embracing a more integrated approach, where elements of cure-focused care and palliative care are delivered concurrently, thus ensuring consistency of care throughout a child's illness and life (Michelson and Steinhorn 2007).

KEY POINT

Palliative care for children should begin at diagnosis, even if cure is a possibility.

As models of care continue to evolve and develop, the child and family must remain central and an integrated approach appears to be essential. Future developments must also involve all agencies working together in the planning and commissioning of services. Given the multiple needs and range of services, integration and co-ordination remain the challenge.

Distinct differences

Although the fundamentals of palliative care can be applied across the age span (Sourkes *et al.* 2005) a number of key differences exist which ultimately affect the provision of care to the child and family (Hynson *et al.* 2003) (see Figure 1.3).

While family involvement is recognized and valued in adult palliative care, it appears to have a much higher profile when caring for children and their families (Price *et al.* 2005). The death of a child presents a major challenge to family relationships (Rando 1983, Raphael 1994), undoubtedly causes major disruption to the immediate family's various subsystems (Davies *et al.* 2004) and renders the

---

Palliative care for children is different for a variety of reasons

Care needs to embrace the whole family.
Holistic care must address the educational needs of the child.
Illnesses rendering need for palliative care are specific and wide-ranging in children.
Length of time of palliative care requirement can be longer in children.
Development emotional, physical and cognitive is continuous in childhood, affecting communication.
Rare illnesses in childhood may be familial and may affect more than one child in the family.
Evidence base underpinning practice is limited.
Numbers of children requiring palliative care are smaller.

Figure 1.3 The uniqueness of children's palliative care

Source: Price *et al.* (2005). Reproduced with kind permission of the *International Journal of Palliative Nursing*.

family and the marital unit notably vulnerable (Riches and Dawson 1996). Care packages, while promoting family functioning, must embrace the whole family (Kenyon and Barnett 2001). A two-way process, where information is shared, is crucial to ensure that families impart their unique knowledge about their child to the interdisciplinary team, and receive information from the team to empower them to make decisions with or on behalf of their child. Sourkes *et al.* (2005: 371) describe sibling relationships as 'a crucial axis in the family', and it is essential to recognize that siblings too are pivotal to the family-centred approach to care at the different stages of the palliative care 'journey'.

Children with life-limiting illness continue to grow and develop emotionally, physically and cognitively throughout their illness trajectory (Price *et al.* 2005). This clearly has an affect on the child's understanding and awareness of their illness and death, ability to be involved in the decision-making process as well as their ever-changing medical and social needs. Schooling and educational needs are essential within the holistic approach to care, not only to ensure that the child learns, but also to forge important social relationships and promote an element of normality (Bouffet *et al.* 1997). Unlike the situation with adult palliative care, where the focus is mainly on patients with malignant diseases, children present with a broad diagnostic mix of conditions that are often prolonged, unpredictable and possibly lead to a more complex disease trajectory (ACT 2003). The hetero-geneity of the illness leads to a need for the involvement by many professional disciplines (Price *et al.* 2005). Furthermore, given the unpredictable nature of the illness trajectory, children with life-limited illness and their families may require palliative care services for a protracted period, often for many years (Rallison and Moules 2004) often intermittently throughout their lives. The inclusion of respite care as part of the care package is therefore important (this topic will be discussed in Chapter 6).

Given the genetic nature of many of the illnesses that mean a child needs a pal-liative care approach, there may be more than one child in a family with the same life-limiting condition. This in turn has an effect on family need and the way in which a family copes (Price *et al.* 2005).

The numbers of children requiring palliative care are smaller than for their adult counterparts, and as a result of this the evidence base underpinning care delivery is more limited than for the adult population. While the current govern-ance agenda demands that care is based on the best possible evidence, the lack of research within children's palliative care has been highlighted (Cooley *et al.* 2000, Institute of Medicine 2002, Emond and Eaton 2004). While the research base has increased in recent years alongside service provision (ACT 2003, 2004), in fact research within this area can be problematic (see Chapter 11).

Specific challenges

Despite the proliferation and increasing recognition of the needs of children requiring a palliative approach, a number of challenging issues have become apparent when developing services and providing care to both children and families (Price *et al.* 2005, Liben *et al.* 2008).

━━━━━━━━━━━━━━━━ **ACTIVITY** ━━━━━━━━━━━━━━━━

Consider the challenges you encounter when caring for children requiring palliative care, and their families.

Some of these challenges summarized in Figure 1.4.

Symptom management/pharmacological issues.
Psychological support for children and families.
Ethical issues: dilemmas in practice and research.
Complex communication issues.
Interdisciplinary team-working.
Fragmentation of services/variance in availability.
Initiating end-of-life care.
Coping strategies for staff stress.

Figure 1.4 Specific challenges in children's palliative care

In a review offering guidance on the commissioning of children's palliative care services (DH 2005), community-led palliative care was identified as being essential to the provision of care for both children and families. Despite this and other recommendations aimed at guiding the organization and delivery of palliative care for children (ACT 1997, 2003, Craft and Killen 2007, DH 2008), however, fragmentation and variance in the availability of services between areas and geographical locations still exist. Ensuring that all children have access to equitable service provision and palliative care continues to prove challenging, and ways of taking services forward will be examined in the final chapter of this book.

Conclusion

While major advances and developments have occurred in recent years in care provision for children requiring palliative care, and their families, this has not been without problems or challenges. The recognition that the needs of such children are unparalleled is widely accepted, and this 'unique way of caring' has now become established across the globe.

These children and their families face a difficult journey along a trajectory of uncertainty. Health and social care professionals working within this 'new interdisciplinary frontier' (Sourkes, *et al.* 2005: 305) have a responsibility to ensure the child and family receive a holistic, flexible care package, delivered within a partnership approach. Care should also be tailored very specifically to individualized and ever-changing needs. As this field of practice continues to grow and develop, further strategic development and continued partnership with children and families is required. The interdisciplinary team caring for children and their families need to ensure that they remain alert to changing needs, are flexible, address the challenges, and ensure that best practice is underpinned by research, education and knowledge.

In the remaining chapters of this book, the health and social care professional will be encouraged to consider these challenges and examine how the provision of comprehensive palliative care can be achieved for children and their families both now and in the future.

Key resources

ACT and RCPCH (Association for Children with Life-threatening or Terminal Conditions and their Families, and Royal College of Paediatrics and Child Health) (2003) *A Guide to the Development of Children's Palliative Care Services* (2nd edn). Bristol: ACT.

Liben, S., Papadatou, D. and Wolfe, J. (2008) Paediatric palliative care: challenges and emerging ideas. *The Lancet* **371**(9615): 852–64.

Worswick, J. (2000) *A House Called Helen: The Development of Hospice Care for Children*. Oxford University Press.

CHAPTER SUMMARY

- Palliative care for children and their families is now recognized as a small but distinct area of practice.

- Palliative Care for children has evolved from the hospice movement and is delivered in a variety of places.

- The philosophy of palliative care is delivered within a partnership of caring, addressing the individual needs of the child and family.

- Care and services for children are different from those for adults in a number of ways.

- Caring for children who have a limited life span is not without its challenges.

- As the speciality develops further, the need for a more substantive research base to underpin practice is essential.

Acknowledgements

Dr Joanne Jordan, School of Nursing and Midwifery, Queen's University, Belfast, for encouragement and support with this chapter.

References

ACT and RCPCH (Association for Children with Life-Threatening or Terminal Conditions and their Families, and Royal College of Paediatrics and Child Health) (1997) *A Guide to the Development of Children's Palliative Care Services*. Bristol: ACT.

ACT and RCPCH (Association for Children with Life-Threatening or Terminal Conditions and their Families, and Royal College of Paediatrics and Child Health) (2003) *A Guide to the Development of Children's Palliative Care Services* (2nd edn). Bristol: ACT.

ACT (Association for Children with Life-Threatening or Terminal Conditions and their Families) (2004) *A Framework for the Development of Integrated Multi-Agency Care Pathways for Children with Life-threatening and Life-limiting Conditions.* Bristol: ACT.

ACT (Association for Children's Palliative Care) (2007a) *Children's Palliative Care and Adult Palliative Care: Similarities and Differences.* Available at: www.act.co.uk

ACT (Association for Children's Palliative Care) (2007b) *The Transition Care Pathway: A Framework for the Development of Integrated Multi-Agency Care Pathways for Young People with Life-threatening and Life-limiting Conditions.* Bristol: ACT.

Bartell, A. and Kissane, D. (2005) Issues in pediatric palliative care: understanding families. *Journal of Palliative Care*, **21**(3): 165–72.

Bignold, S., Ball, S. and Cribb, A. (1994) *Nursing Families with Children with Cancer: The Work of the Paediatric Oncology Outreach Nurse Specialists.* London; Kings College.

Bouffet, E., Zucchinelli, V., Costanzo, P. and Blanchard, P. (1997) Schooling as part of palliative care in paediatric oncology. *Palliative Medicine* **11**: 133–9.

Children's Hospices UK (2008) *About Children's Hospice Services.* Available at: www.childhospice.org.uk/page.asp?section=30&sectionTitle=About+children%27s+hospice+services; accessed 20 October 2008.

Children's Palliative Care Alliance (2008) *Welcome for New Strategy to Help Life-limited Children,* Press release, 19 February. Available at: www.act.org.uk

Cooley, C., Adeodu, S., Aldred, H., Beesley, S., Leung, A. and Thacker, L. (2000) Paediatric palliative care: a lack of research-based evidence. *International Journal of Palliative Nursing* **6**(7): 346–51.

Craft, A. and Killen, S. (2007) *Palliative Care Services for Children and Young People in England.* Available at: www.dh.gov.uk/en/Publicationsandstatistics/Publications/PublicationsPolicyandGuidance/DH_074459.

Davies, B., Gudmundsdottir, M., Worden, B., Orloff, S., Sumner, L. and Brenner, P. (2004) 'Living in the dragon's shadow': fathers' experiences of a child's life-limiting illness. Death Studies **28**: 111–35.

Davies, R. E. (1999) The Diana community nursing team and paediatric palliative care. *British Journal of Nursing* **8**(8): 506, 508–11.

DH (Department of Health) (2005) *Commissioning Children's and Young People's Palliative Care Services. A Practical Guide for the NHS Commissioners.* London: Department of Health.

DH (Department of Health) (2008) *Better Lives: Better Care. Improving outcomes and experiences for children, young people and their families living with life-limiting and life threatening conditions.* London: Department of Health.

DHSSPS (Department of Health, Social Services and Public Safety) and University of Ulster (2007) *Complex Needs: The Nursing Response to Children and Young People with Complex Physical Healthcare Needs.* Belfast: DHSSPS.

Downing, J. (2008) Children's palliative care: thinking outside the box. *International Journal of Palliative Nursing* **14**(5): 212.

Emond, A. and Eaton, N. (2004) Supporting children with complex healthcare needs and their families – an overview of the research agenda. *Child Care, Health and Development* **30**: 195–9.

Farrell, M. and Sutherland, P. (1998) Providing paediatric palliative care: collaboration in practice. *British Journal of Nursing* **7**(12): 712–16.

Feudtner, C. (2007) Collaborative communication in pediatric palliative care: a foundation for problem-solving and decision making. *Pediatrics Clinic of North America* **54**: 593–607.

Glare, P. and Virik, K. (2001) Can we do better in end of life care? The mixed management model of palliative care. *Medical Journal of Australia* **175**: 530–6.

Goldman, A. (1998) ABC of palliative care – special problems of children. *British Medical Journal* **316**: 49–52.

Goldman, A. (2007) An overview of paediatric palliative care. *Medical Principles in Practice,* **16**: 46–7.

Goldman, A., Beardsmore, S. and Hunt, J. (1990) Palliative care for children with cancer – home, hospital or hospice? *Archives of Disease in Childhood* **65**: 641–3.

Hain, R. and Wallace , A. (2008) Progress in palliative care for children. *Pediatrics and Child Health,* **18**(3): 141–6.

Hewitt-Taylor, J. (2005) Caring for children with complex and continuing health care needs. *Nursing Standard* **19**(42): 41–7.

Himelstein, B. P., Hilden, J. M., Boldt, A. M. and Weissman, D. (2004) Pediatric palliative care. *New England Journal of Medicine* **350**: 1752–62.

Howell, D. A. (1995) Special services for children. In: Doyle, D., Hanks, G. and Macdonald, N. (eds) *Oxford Textbook of Palliative Medicine.* Oxford University Press.

Hutchinson, F., King, N. and Hain, R. (2003) Terminal care in paediatrics: where we are now. *Postgraduate Medical Journal* **79**: 566–68.

Hynson, J., Gillis, J., Collins, J., Irving, H. and Trethewie, J. (2003) The dying child: how is care different? *Medical Journal of Australia* **179**: S20–22.

ICPCN (International Children's Palliative Care Network (2007) *The Need for Children's Palliative Care.* Available at: www.icpcn.org.uk; accessed on 21 October 2008.

ICPCN (International Children's Palliative Care Network (2008) *The ICPCN Charter.* Available at: www.act.org.uk/dmdocuments/ICPCN%20Charter.pdf; accessed on 23 October 2008.

IOM (Institute of Medicine) (2002) *When Children Die: Improving Palliative and End-of-life Care for Children and Families.* Washington, DC: National Academy Press.

Kenyon, E. and Barnett, N. (2001) Partnership in nursing care: the Blackburn model. *Journal of Child Health Care* **5**(1): 35–8.

Lamers, W. M. (2002) Defining hospice and palliative care: some further thoughts. *Journal of Pain and Palliative Care Pharmacotherapy* **16**(3): 65–71.

Lauer, M. E. and Camitta, B, M. (1980) Home care for dying children: a nursing model. *Pediatrics* **97**: 1032–5.

Lenton, S., Goldman, A., Eaton, N. and Southall, D. (2006) Development and epidemiology. In Goldman, A., Hain, R. and Liben, S. (2006) *Oxford Textbook of Palliative Care for Children.* Oxford: Oxford University Press.

Liben, S., Papadatou, D. and Wolfe, J. (2008) Paediatric palliative care: challenges and emerging ideas. *The Lancet* **371**(9615): 852–64.

McCready Donnelly Lowry (2007) *Evaluation of the Partnership Arrangements for the Delivery of a Children's Hospice at Home Service in the Western Board.* Magherafelt: McCready Donnelly Lowry Ltd.

McCulloch, R., Comac, M. and Craig, F. (2008) Paediatric palliative care: Coming of age in oncology? *European Journal of Cancer* **44**(8):1139–45.

McNeilly, P., Price, J. and McCloskey, S. (2004) The use of syringe drivers: a paediatric perspective. *International Journal of Palliative Nursing* **10**(8): 399–403.

McNeilly, P. and Price, J. (2007) Interdisciplinary teamworking in paediatric palliative care. *European Journal of Palliative Care* **14**(2): 64–7.

Michelson, K. N. and Steinhorn, D. M. (2007) Pediatric end-of-life issues and palliative care. *Clinical Pediatric Emergency Medicine* **8**: 212–19.

NICE (National Institute for Health and Clinical Excellence) (2005) *Improving Outcomes in Children and Young People with Cancer.* Available at: www.nice.org.uk

Nicholl, H. (2007) An investigation of the terminology used for children with life-limiting conditions. *Journal of Children and Young People's Nursing* **1**(3): 137–41.

Pfund, R. (2007) *Palliative Care Nursing of Children and Young People.* Oxford: Radcliffe Publishing.

Price, J. and Spence, N. (2004) Play in the community – quality care for the child with cancer. *Cancer Nursing Practice* **38**: 31–4.

Price, J., McNeilly, P. and McFarlane, M. (2005) Paediatric palliative care in the UK: past, present and future. *International Journal of Palliative Nursing* **11**(3): 124–9.

Rallison, L., Limachev, L. H., Clinton, M. (2006) Future echoes in pediatric palliative care: becoming sensitive to language. *Journal of Palliative Care*, **22**(2): 99–104.

Rallison, L. and Moules, N. (2004) The unspeakable nature of pediatric palliative care: unveiling many cloaks. *Journal of Family Nursing* **10**(3): 287–301.

Rando, T. (1983) An investigation of grief and adaptation in parents whose children have died from cancer. *Journal of Pediatric Psychology* **8**: 3–19.

Raphael, B. (1994) *The Anatomy of Bereavement*. London: Hutchinson.

Riches, G. and Dawson, P. (1996) An intimate loneliness: evaluating the impact of a child's death on parental self-identity and marital relationships. *Journal of Family Therapy* **18**: 1–22.

Sourkes, B., Frankel, L., Brown, M., Contro, N., Benitz, W., Case, C., Good, J., Jones, L., Komejan, J., Modderman-Marshall, J., Reichard, W., Sentivany-Collins, S. and Sunde, C. (2005) Food, toys and love: pediatric palliative care. *Current Problems in Pediatric Aadolescent Health* Care **35**: 350–86.

Steele, R. (2000) Trajectory of certain death at an unknown time with degenerative life-threatening illness. *Cancer Journal of Nursing Research* **32**: 49–67.

Steele, R., Deman, S., Cadell, S., Davies, B., Siden, H. and Straatman, L. (2008) Families' transition to a Canadian paediatric hospice: Part 1 planning a pilot study. *International Journal of Palliative Nursing* **14**(5): 248–56.

UNCRC (United Nations Convention on the Rights of the Child) (1989) UNICEF Geneva. Available at: www.unicef.org/crc/crc.htm; accessed 21 October 2008.

Vickers, J., Thompson, A., Collins, G. S., Childs, M. and Hain, R. (2007) Place and provision of palliative care for children with progressive cancer: a study by the Paediatric Oncology Nurses' Forum/United Kingdom Children's Cancer Study Group Palliative Care Working Group. *Journal of Clinical Oncology* **25**(28): 4472–6.

WMPMT (West Midlands Paediatric Macmillan Team) (2005) *Palliative Care for Children with Malignant Disease*. London: Quay Books.

Worswick, J. (2000) A House Called Helen: *The Development of Hospice Care for Children*. Oxford University Press.

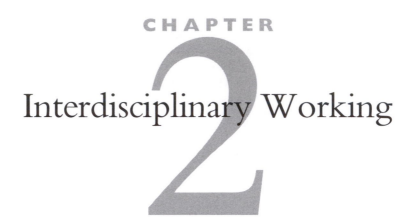

CHAPTER 2

Interdisciplinary Working

Patricia McNeilly and Frances Gilmore

Introduction

Successful interdisciplinary teamwork is a fundamental part of health care, and is perhaps one that is commonly taken for granted. The ability to work as part of a team is a necessary attribute for entry into the health care professions (General Medical Council 2003, Nursing and Midwifery Council 2004), but there is a lack of ongoing evaluation concerning how individuals work effectively as part of such a team. As discussed in the first chapter of this book, ACT outlined the key principles of children's palliative care, including the notion that the delivery of care should be 'well co-ordinated, with an emphasis on continuity of services' (ACT, 2004: 9). However, as Jassal and Sims (2006) and Speck (2006) point out, effective teams do not just occur. Rather, they need active nurturing and management in order to be effective. The purpose of this chapter is to unravel the complexities of team- working within paediatric palliative care, discuss the challenges inherent in caring for life-limited children and their families within the team context, and explore how team-working may be improved within this domain of practice. Recognizing the importance of interdisciplinary team-working, various government bodies and key agencies have produced a number of national and international policy documents that further highlight the importance of this issue for children and their families.

KEY POINT

Effective teams do not just occur; they need active nurturing and management in order to be productive.

Policy context

In recent years, there has been a shift from the traditional top–down approach to a more collaborative way of working with children and young people. This has been facilitated to some extent by the increase in the provision of community services caring for children in their own homes (DH 2006). The growing input from professionals from various settings, including the voluntary sector, together with the need for children's services to be provided in or near their own homes has increased the need for effective team-working across professional, geographical and organizational boundaries. However, findings from the recent review of children's palliative care services in England (Craft and Killen 2007), suggest that there is little evidence of the health, education, social care and voluntary services working together.

Numerous policy and strategic documents support the notion that the key to future service development is the need for professionals to work in a more integrated manner around the needs of children and their families (McNeilly and Price 2007). Both the Kennedy and Laming reports pointed towards poor co-ordination and communication between services as key elements of the failure to provide optimal levels of care and protection for children and young people (RCPCH 2006). Subsequently, many recommendations and standards have been established in the wake of the government's 'Every Child Matters' agenda. The National Service Frameworks have been instrumental in blueprinting a set of standards for children with complex and longer- term health needs, including those requiring palliative care. Within Standard 8, which addresses the needs of these children, it is recognized that a cohesive, co-ordinated approach is required between health, social care and education (DfES and DH 2004a). In order to achieve such an approach, a number of Common Core Skills have been developed for the children's workforce including a particular emphasis on multi-agency working and the sharing of information (DfES 2005). Such skills include the need for role clarity in addition to developing an increasing understanding of the roles of others in relation to varying professional standards, organizational issues and ways of working. Most recently, in 2006, a Children's Workforce Network (comprising eleven national agencies from various sectors of the children's workforce) was set up within the UK in order to further promote joined-up services for children, young people and their families within the UK, and work is ongoing in this regard. One such project is a move towards an Integrated Qualifications Network (IQF) for those working with children and young people, and the proposal of a set of values concerning inter-professional work with colleagues. Central to these values is the fostering of respect for the expertise of others, together with the knowledge that both professionals and families value transparency and reliability. The need for children's practitioners to be supportive of each other is also highlighted. While these values have been developed from a generalist perspective, they are arguably of particular importance in the children's palliative care team.

What is a team?

Given the diversity of organizational teams, it is not surprising that there is no consensus around what constitutes a team. Payne (2000) provides a comprehensive review of definitions of teams and teamwork within interdisciplinary care. Included is a definition by Pritchard and Pritchard (1994: 13), who claim that a team is 'a group of people who make different contributions towards the same goal'. Similarly, Partridge (2007: 2) maintains that a team 'combines the energy, motivation, experiences and expertise of individuals for a shared purpose so that the team achieves more than the sum of its parts'. Regardless of which definition one uses, a central concept within the definitions of teams concerns a common aim goal, task or outcome. It is widely accepted that teamwork has three main components: namely, the task (what the team is to achieve); the individuals (the members of the team); and the team itself (the dynamics within the team) (Partridge 2007). It is often assumed that teams generally function in a co-operative manner (Cott 1998), though this may not always be the case. Given the number of 'teams' or groups an individual may be a member of, from both a personal and professional perspective, it is not surprising that each team member comes to the interdisciplinary team with varying sets of values, which form the basis of teamwork. According to Speck (2006), ascribing to a set of shared *team values* avoids potential conflicts with personal values. Speck suggests that team values within palliative care should include those set out in Figure 2.1. In terms of paediatric palliative care, a central value concerns the acknowledgement that the needs of the child and family should remain a pivotal issue.

═══════════════════ **ACTIVITY** ═══════════════════

Reflect on the number of teams or groups of which you are a member, both personally and professionally, and the values of each team.

- The child and family's needs should come first.

- 'The importance of *working together* to achieve the aim' (Speck, 2006: 4) is paramount; that is, if something goes wrong, the whole team is examined, not the individual involved.

- Each team member is respected and valued, regardless of his/her role.

- Open and honest communication is valued.

- There should be open access to information; information should not be withheld as a means of disempowering others

Figure 2.1   Values of the palliative care team.

Source: Speck (2006).

As Firth–Cozens (2001) points out, health care team members are unique because of their obligations towards various professional bodies as well as to the team itself. As a consequence, this can 'muddy the waters' in relation to allegiance towards and performance of the interdisciplinary team. Such diversity in teams can at times be a challenging issue, but it is generally accepted that team members with varying professional, personal and cultural backgrounds can be of benefit, in terms of understanding and meeting the needs of their clients, in this case the child and family. Furthermore, in a diverse team, problem-solving and decision-making tends to be more creative (Partridge 2007). A number of myths about teamwork exist and are worth bearing in mind in relation to paediatric palliative care teams. These include the notion that decisions must be made by consensus, and that individuals will eventually become an effective team simply by working together (Hawryluck and Ryan 2001). In fact, decisions are rarely made with the agreement of all, and working together in itself does not produce effective outcomes for teams, a point we shall return to later.

The health care team

There are numerous terms used to describe or refer to the health care team, and these are often used interchangeably without much consideration. Traditionally, the term multi-disciplinary was used to describe various professionals involved with the child and family (McNeilly and Price 2007), and indeed this is still often the case. However, more recently, a number of alternative terminologies have been adopted as a means of better capturing the relationships and functions within the health care team of today. While the term 'multi-disciplinary' suggests the lone working of professionals with differing roles and little co-ordination (Watson *et al.* 2002), the alternative term 'interdisciplinary' working implies active communication in terms of information sharing and working together. In the latter situation, it is anticipated that the sum of the team is greater than its parts (Speck 2006). In relation to paediatric palliative care, this approach has developed and evolved in recent years. A useful working definition of interdisciplinary health care team is provided by Drinka and Clark who suggest that it 'integrates a group of individuals with diverse training and backgrounds who work together as an identified unit or system. Team members consistently collaborate to solve patient problems that are too complex to be solved by one discipline or many disciplines in sequence' (2000: 6).

Given the variation in operational definitions of teams, interdisciplinary teams and modes of team-working within health care, how then might the children's palliative care team be defined? One possible definition is that it is a diverse group of individuals from various settings who work flexibly across professional and organizational boundaries, and who collectively and collaboratively aim to provide holistic care for children with palliative care needs and their families. A partnership approach to this care is paramount, both within the team and with the child and family.

KEY POINT

The children's palliative care team may be defined as a diverse group of individuals from various settings who work flexibly across professional and organizational boundaries, and who collectively and collaboratively aim to provide holistic care for children with palliative care needs and their families. A partnership approach to this care is paramount, both within the team and with the child and family.

The children's palliative care team

The children's palliative care team is unique in a number of ways, not least because of the potentially large numbers of professionals and agencies that may be involved with the child and family. A number of models of care delivery operate within the UK; these were highlighted in Chapter 1. Clearly, models of care have a direct impact on how the team operates and communicates, not only between themselves but also with the child and family. An example of those who may be involved is included in Figure 2.2, though in many cases there are considerably more or fewer people, as desired by the family. At times, depending on the health of the child, input from professionals may be great and at other times much less. One of the skills of working in such a team is to recognize intuitively when input should be increased or reduced, in discussion with the child and family.

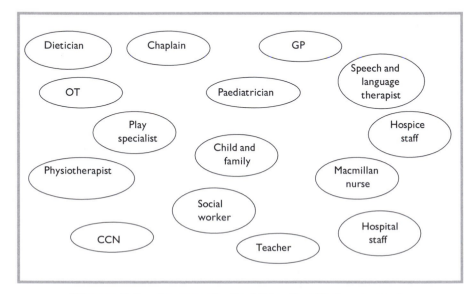

Figure 2.2   An example of a children's palliative care team

Source: McNeilly and Price (2007: 65). Reproduced with the kind permission of the *European Journal of Palliative Care*.

Parents as members of the team

Parents of children with life-limiting and life-threatening conditions are considered to be experts in their child's care and they develop many complex skills in order to meet their child's needs (Warr 2007). This being the case, they are undisputedly pivotal members of the paediatric palliative care team. Despite the ongoing acceptance of the philosophy of partnership working and family- centred care, findings of research indicate that this is not always the case in practice. For example, in her research with families whose children experienced a prolonged death, Steele (2002) reported that parents sometimes found that professionals were reticent about parental involvement. Furthermore, some parents found that care was regimented rather than family-centred and individualized. Clearly, there is a great need to find a balance between helping parents to participate in and maintain control over the care of their child and providing support when it is needed. Open lines of communication, such as those explored in Chapter 3, are a key issue in assessing and responding to individual families' needs. All members of the team, including the children and their parents, should share the same goals, and parents should maintain ownership of the care that their child receives. Suggestions as to how to achieve this are set out in Figure 2.3. Goals should be negotiated between the child and parents, and other team members.

Benefits of team-working

Operationally defining and providing evidence for the effectiveness of palliative care teams is a contentious and challenging issue. Indeed, as Sloper (2004) points out, there is a paucity of evidence concerning the effectiveness of inter-agency working in terms of providing optimal care for children and young people. However, it is generally accepted that successful team-working has positive benefits for those requiring palliative care (Crawford and Price 2003) as well as for health

---

- Remember, first and foremost, that the child and parents are experts in the care of the child.

- Share and exchange information with the child and family at an appropriate level.

- Discuss and negotiate goals of care using a partnership approach.

- Be aware that your input may not be required on an ongoing basis, particularly if the child's condition is fairly stable.

- Avoid making assumptions, they may not b e correct – ask and check your understanding of what is conveyed.

- Encourage questions and provide honest answers.

- Ask the child/parents if there is anything else they want to happen.

Figure 2.3   Ensuring that the child and family maintain ownership of their care

care professionals (Abbott *et al.* 2005). Anecdotal evidence suggests that team-working promotes positive outcomes for both the patients and the professionals themselves. Such benefits for patients requiring palliative care have included an improvement in physical symptoms (Jack *et al.* 2004) and quality of life (Schrader *et al.* 2002). Benefits for practitioners working with children have included increased job satisfaction and personal development (Abbott *et al.* 2005). Mutual support between members has also been identified as an advantage of working within the palliative care team (Crawford and Price 2003).

The nature and dynamics of the children's palliative care team

Like any team, health care teams are influenced by a wide variety of psychological group processes and, according to O'Connor *et al.* (2006), psychological factors on an individual level – for example, personality variables – can also have a signifi-cant impact on the effectiveness of the palliative care team. Historically, the stages of team development, as first described by Tuckman (1965), have been used to describe the formation and reformation of teams, and these are still frequently used today (see Figure 2.4). They represent a healthy and inevitable process that was evidenced during the early proliferation of paediatric palliative care services. Each stage is associated with specific characteristics – though, as Payne (2000) points out, it was not devised to take into account alterations in team dynamics when individuals come and go, a common occurrence in the health care setting.

The first stage listed in Figure 2.4, forming, refers to early team development when team members are trying to establish how they fit into the group and exploring potential ways of working. Following this initial 'forming', a period of 'storming' occurs, where members try to establish how the group might best operate in order to achieve its goals. This stage is commonly characterized by con-flict, as individuals challenge the views of others within the group. Next comes a period of 'norming', in which ways of working become established, and while there is still some disagreement, the team starts to function in a more positive manner (Partridge 2007). This stage is also characterized by mutual support between team members, which can be instrumental in the progression towards the stage of 'performing', when the team operates effectively in terms of attaining their goals. Applying this to the delivery of palliative care, Hawryluck and Ryan

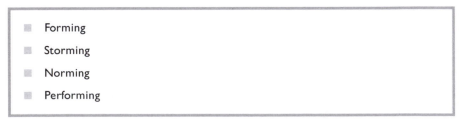

- Forming
- Storming
- Norming
- Performing

Figure 2.4 The stages of team development
Source: Tuckman (1965).

(2001) propose a further stage of 'reforming' that occurs when team dynamics are altered; for example, when a team member leaves or a new one joins. During this stage, team development may regress to an earlier stage, and so the process is constantly changing.

=========================== **ACTIVITY** ===========================

Consider the dynamics of your team. What happens when someone leaves or a new person joins the team?

The challenges of team-working in children's palliative care

Working as part of the children's palliative care team is without doubt challenging. Such challenges arise from a number of issues, including the size of the team, leadership of the team, potential conflict, role ambiguity and the blurring or crossing of boundaries, all of which are discussed in the following sections.

Size of the team

One of the challenges of team-working within this area concerns the potentially large number of people involved with the child and family. It is estimated that children and young people with complex health needs have contact with approximately ten different professionals and make twenty visits per year to clinics/hospitals (DfES and DH 2004b). For others, including those with palliative care needs, these figures are multiplied. Also unique to the care of children is the added issue of addressing their ongoing educational needs, necessitating an inclusive approach between education and health care. The complexities of such team-working may lead not only to difficulties in communication and the sharing of information, but also to increase the opportunity for conflicting information to be given, which is particularly stressful for parents. This is compounded by the lengthy time frame over which care is provided in some cases and, as such, it is inevitable that some staff leave and are replaced. This can be challenging for the team in terms of assisting a new staff member to settle in, but also for the family, who have to get to know and learn to trust someone all over again. Clearly, communication and support mechanisms within the team are key if such issues are to be kept to a minimum.

Leadership in the paediatric palliative care team

In any team, individuals strive for personal recognition of their work and this is a normal process. An inevitable outcome of this is the development of power struggles (Hawryluck and Ryan 2001), and this can be problematic if not resolved quickly. One way of avoiding such struggles is the clear identification of a leader and a clear structure of accountability, as power should not be distributed equally within the team. Previous research concerning adult palliative teams indicates that the leadership role is unclear within this specialty (Hill 1998), though it is normally physician- led, and Hill's research in1998 demonstrated that nurses are happy for doctors to take the lead. The situation is perhaps more complex in children's palliative care as, during periods of good health, the child's key worker in the community may take on the leadership role for a period of time.

Furthermore, as O'Connor *et al.* (2006) point out, while the team leader is commonly assumed to be the doctor or nurse (O'Connor *et al.* 2006), there is no reason why this should not be an allied health professional or a social worker however, this would seldom be the case. Dominant personalities may be also be problematic where leadership is concerned (Crawford and Price 2003), though thankfully this is rarely the case within this specialty. One way of resolving leadership issues within the children's palliative care team is to foster an ethos of open communication and revisiting accountability within the team on an ongoing basis.

Conflict in teamwork

A certain amount of conflict is an inevitable part of team development, for some of the reasons mentioned above. On a positive note, in a research study by Hill (1998) on multi-professional teamwork, the concept of conflict was not raised by many participants, and those who did felt that it was inevitable rather than problematic. Indeed, it is widely accepted that disagreements and discussions around decision-making are a constructive and positive facet of ongoing, optimal team-working (Partridge 2007). Similarly, it is also acknowledged that, for a team to be effective, a diverse range of personalities and learning styles should be represented. Partridge (2007) points out that if everyone on the team always agreed decisions without any discussion or debate, then the social-psychological process of 'groupthink' would be in operation. Groupthink occurs when group harmony and the avoidance of dissent becomes more important than the decisions being made (Myers 2008). Members of the children's palliative care team must feel free to express their ideas and opinions and have their voice heard, with the interests of the child and family firmly at the heart of the matter. Speck (2006) suggests that conflict or problems associated with team dynamics may be addressed during individual and group supervision sessions, although this might be difficult in the community setting, where team members are spread out geographically. Stress at individual, team or organizational level may increase the potential for conflict within the team, so open, honest communication, supervision and peer support is vital.

When acknowledged and resolved, conflicts can help the team to function more effectively and cohesively. While we deal with conflict in a number of ways, Partridge (2007) maintains that collaboration is the most successful strategy; that is, both (or all) parties should work on a task together to promote joint problem-solving. While there may be disagreement or conflict, if each team member is valued as suggested in Figure 2.1 above, and there is an ethos of open communication, then it should be possible to achieve a successful resolution if it is handled constructively, and this is often the case. However, a number of additional issues can alter the dynamic within the palliative care team – for example, role ambiguity – and these can also have an impact on care delivery.

Role ambiguity

Role ambiguity can be particularly problematic in palliative care because of the holistic nature of care (Sealey and Feuer, 2007) that is negotiated with the family. Role ambiguity occurs when individuals lack clarity about their role (Luthans 2002). Previous research has demonstrated that professionals working within palliative care have a lack of understanding of the roles of others, and this can lead to unintentional 'gatekeeping' whereby individuals do not get the full package of support that they may require (Bliss *et al.* 2000). While elements of differing professionals' roles are clear-cut – for example, in relation to physical care or symptom management – many professionals contribute to the psycho-social support of the child and family, deeming it a 'shared realm' (O'Connor *et al.* 2006: 5). For example, the GP, the paediatrician, the Macmillan or hospice nurse, the community children's nurse or the social worker may all provide bereavement care, but whose role is it? Nurses seem to have the greatest difficulty with role ambiguity. In a study of hospital palliative teams by Hill (1998), nurses found it particularly difficult to define their role clearly, whereas medical staff and social workers had no difficulty.

A key issue in terms of involvement of professionals or others with the child and family is successful partnership working, not only between the team members, but also between those involved and the child and family. It is imperative that the child and family control who is involved and the nature of their input at any given time. Recognizing that most people working within health and social care (and in particular children's palliative care) are there because they want to make a difference, regardless of their role, can have a positive and unifying effect on the team (Benson and Rice 2007).

=========================== **ACTIVITY** ===========================

Think of three individuals with whom you work. Write down five key features of their role in caring for children with palliative care needs. How difficult did you find this?

Blurring and crossing the boundaries

A similar issue arises around the so-called blurring of boundaries which, according to some, is desirable in palliative care (see Hill 1998) in order to ensure flexible and optimal service provision (DH 2008). For others, however, it can be a source of stress. As O'Connor *et al.* (2006) point out, without clearly defined roles and boundaries, palliative care professionals may become unsure of the value of their place in the team. There is some disagreement within the literature around 'blurring' and 'crossing' of boundaries. This is to some extent clarified by Rushmer (2005), who explored and clarified the complexities around this aspect of interdisciplinary working. She maintained that the notion of blurred boundaries can lead to mistrust and resentment, and suggested that the opposite is required; that is, clear, specific and negotiated boundaries that remain a fundamental part of integrated working practices. In terms of palliative care, this means that while there may be shared areas of care between professionals, there is equal emphasis and respect for areas that are specific to an individual's role and are therefore not to be shared. In short, Rushmer refuted the notion of 'blurred boundaries' and maintained that boundaries may be 'crossed' unavoidably on occasion, but this situation is acceptable so long as it is discussed and negotiated later with those involved:

> A blurred boundary is imprecision about who does what when ... A crossed boundary (as the name suggests) is the crossing of a boundary that does exist. In everyday life, sometimes boundaries are crossed with permission; at other times, boundaries are violated without consent (Rushmer 2005: 81).

Good working relationships within the team, that foster open communication, promotes opportunities to negotiate and discuss differing roles within the team.

FURTHER READING

Read Rushmer, R. (2005) Blurred boundaries damage inter-professional working. *Nurse Researcher* 12(3): 74–85 and reflect on the boundaries in your own team.

ACTIVITY

Consider the challenges of your own team and identify how these could be addressed.

Care-co-ordination schemes

A number of initiatives have been developed over recent years as a means of enhancing teamwork. Parents have also become more involved in the development and ongoing delivery of such schemes for disabled children, including those requiring palliative care across the UK (Greco and Sloper 2004). Such schemes include keyworking, 'Team Around the Child' and integrated 'care pathways'.

Keyworking

The key worker concept for children with varying levels of health and social care need has been a recurring recommendation in social and health care policy since the mid-1970s (Court Report 1976, Children Act 1989). More recently, it has been advocated strongly in children's palliative care documents (ACT 2003, Craft and Killen 2007, DH 2008). The National Service Framework for Children Young People and Maternity Services (DfES and DH 2004a: 28) states that:

> 'Parents of severely disabled children or those with high levels of need require a single point of contact with services and an effective, trusted and informed named person (a "key worker") to help them obtain the services they require.'

However, despite such recommendations, it is estimated that up to a third of families still do not have a designated key worker, and others are unclear about the key worker role (Greco *et al.* 2007). Families need a 'knowledgeable doer', an easily accessible person who can be contacted for information and advice;

someone who is there for them on both a practical and an emotional level (Kirk and Glendinning 2004). The key worker acts as a single point of contact for the family and helps them to engage with the many professionals providing care for their child. They also have the necessary skills and knowledge to cross traditional service boundaries to work with other statutory and voluntary agencies, aiming to tailor and co-ordinate services to better meet individual and family needs (Sloper *et al.* 2005). The views of parents are vital in determining the role of the key worker. In an evaluation of the key working process in Warwickshire by Barton and Clarke (2005), parents outlined a number of elements of the key worker role as being important, and these are evident in the case study and role of the Community Children's Nurse presented below.

CLINICAL FOCUS

Jack is a 4-year-old with cerebral palsy who lives with his parents and sisters, aged 6 and 7. Lately, his condition has deteriorated and he has numerous admissions to hospital; he is having increased seizure activity, is more unsettled and is requiring more suction. He has a PEG tube and is enterally fed. His parents are finding it increasingly difficult to cope. He is known to many different professionals from the local hospital, primary care, voluntary sector and education, and currently has regular contact with around eighteen professionals. He is a pupil at the local special school, but recently he has not been well enough to attend as the current support staff are not trained to give him rectal diazepam. His key worker is the Community Children's Nurse, who has known the family since Jack was born.

INTERDISCIPLINARY INSIGHT

The role of the Community Children's Nurse in Jack's care

The Community Children's Nurse, acting as Jack's key worker, will:

- Arrange regular home visits in negotiation with the child and family.
- Assess Jack's needs in partnership with the parents and jointly with relevant members of the interdisciplinary team.
- Be a single point of reference for information and advice, and act as an advocate for the child and family.
- Devise a care plan which addresses Jack's physical, social, emotional and spiritual needs.
- Co-ordinate the input of the various professionals to avoid unnecessary duplication of roles.
- Arrange regular interdisciplinary meetings to review and update the plan of care.
- Arrange for any educational needs of parents and carers to be met, including school staff in relation to administration of appropriate rescue medication.
- Provide information and signposting to other services and agencies as required.
- Provide emotional support and be a listening ear for the family.

Where the key worker system is implemented there are two recognized models of delivery: the non-designated and the designated model (Barton and Clarke 2005). The key worker may be someone already working with the family in a professional capacity, and in addition to this they assume responsibility for co-ordinating the care being delivered. This is known as the *non-designated* model of service provision. The professional is key worker for perhaps two or three children alongside his or her generic caseload. In other areas, key workers are employed specifically for this role and may have responsibility for up to thirty families. This is the second model, the so-called *designated model*, of service provision. Both models were evaluated by Greco *et al.* (2005) and they found advantages and dis-advantages in both. The designated key workers felt they had more time for families, greater knowledge of services, high levels of motivation and a level of independence, which allowed them to advocate effectively for families. Disadvantages included potential loss of skills and the creation of a 'hybrid profession'. Non-designated key workers felt that they brought their experience, skills and knowledge to their work, but cited lack of time, role conflict and role boundaries as disadvantages.

Evaluation of a number of service co-ordination schemes for children with dis-abilities in the UK all illustrate clearly the benefits of the key worker model for the child, the family and the professional (Barton and Clarke, 2005). Key working was found to enable families to have better relationships and partnerships with services. Families reported improvements in services received, and experienced easier access to information about services. In some cases, parents feel empowered to take on the role of key worker themselves. Professionals employed in the key working role have reported greater levels of job satisfaction, greater opportunities for personal development and improved knowledge and skills (Townsley *et al.* 2004). Central to all care co-ordination must be the expressed needs and require-ments of the child and family. Recognition of the expertise that the family will have acquired during their child's illness is an important aspect of effective inter-disciplinary working. One way this can be facilitated is through the deployment of key workers who can 'coordinate, advocate and communicate with, and on behalf of the family' (Jassal and Sims 2006: 519).

KEY POINT

Families need an easily accessible person they can contact for information and advice, someone who is there for them on a practical and emotional level (Kirk and Glendinning 2004).

'Team Around the Child'

A further approach that fosters a joined-up approach is the 'Team Around the Child' (TAC), devised by Peter Limbrick in the 1990's (Limbrick 2004). As its name suggests, the focus of the TAC approach is the central position of the child and family, and the notion that parents are equal members of the team. Lone working by professionals is very much discouraged, and an understanding of the contribution of colleagues is a fundamental aspect of TAC. As Limbrick (2005) points out, a crucial feature of TAC concerns the small number of people involved (three to five), which ensures that the family is not swamped by health care professionals and that their voice is heard. The importance of having a key worker or lead professional is maintained in this system, the benefits of which were discussed in the previous section. However, the key worker cannot work alone and is dependent on identified team members who will provide a holistic package of care, together with the parents and wider family. Therefore, within the TAC approach, the health care professional must have a therapeutic, supportive and working relationship not only with the family, but also with colleagues from a variety of professions and agencies.

Integrated care pathways

The use of integrated care pathways (ICPs) is a further way of facilitating and co-ordinating interdisciplinary and inter-agency care (Davies 2006). The White Paper, *Our Health, Our Care, Our Say* (DH 2006) recommended the further development of care pathways in the light of the shift from acute hospital to primary care settings. Essentially, these pathways set out clearly how best care should be delivered, provide a set of standards against which outcomes may be measured, and promote the sharing of information as a written record. Such single planning and documentation of care by professionals has been ongoing for some time. Until recently, ICPs had mainly been used within the hospital setting for children with specific acute conditions. However, in 2004, ACT produced an all-inclusive ICP for children with life-threatening and life-limiting conditions that crosses the boundary between hospital-based and home care for children. The ICP proposed by ACT is based on the five standards detailed in Figure 2.5. The potential benefits for children and families include better co-ordination of care and improved communication, with less duplication of the care provided, a plan that anticipates the care required, better equality of care between and within regions, and the maintenance of a family- centred approach (ACT 2004).

Work is ongoing in this area; however, initiating change and implementing such frameworks is a challenging issue that takes time and patience. One of the main reasons for this is the complexity of service provision and diverse structures that do not map on to each other (RCPCH 2006). In the early stages of the implementation of ICPs it may be worth considering the advice from the RCPCH (2006: 15): 'It may be better to network some components of the pathway, and succeed, rather than attempt to link all the pathway components and fail.'

ACTIVITY

Consider how the ACT integrated care pathway might be implemented in your area of practice. What stages would be involved?

The first standard
Every family should receive the disclosure of their child's prognosis in a face-to-face discussion in privacy and should be treated with respect, honesty and sensitivity. Information should be provided both for the child and the family in language that they can understand.

The second standard
Every child and family diagnosed in the hospital setting should have an agreed transfer plan involving hospital, community services and the family, and should be provided with the resources they require before leaving hospital.

The third standard
Every family should receive a multi-agency assessment of their needs as soon as possible after diagnosis or recognition, and should have their needs reviewed at appropriate intervals.

The fourth standard
Every child and family should have a multi-agency care plan agreed with them for the delivery of co-ordinated care and support to meet their individual needs. A key worker to assist with this should be identified and agreed with the family.

The fifth standard
Every child and family should be helped to decide on an end of life plan and should be provided with care and support to achieve this as closely as possible.

Figure 2.5 Standards: an integrated care plan for children with
life-threatening and life-limiting conditions
Source: ACT (2004). Reproduced with the kind permission of ACT.

Enhancing the performance of children's palliative care teams

Although many professional bodies emphasize the importance of working within the interdisciplinary team, health care professionals are not actively taught how to operate within a team or deal with potential problems that might arise. This may provide a good starting point if team-working within paediatric palliative care is to be improved. Inter-professional education (IPE) provides an opportunity for students from a variety of professional backgrounds to develop a deeper understanding of the roles of others and a number of specifically designed programmes have been developed (see, for example, Price and McNeilly 2006). Wee *et al.* maintain that IPE in palliative care should start at the undergraduate level, where the 'seeds for interprofessional teamworking need to be sown early' (2001: 488). Wee *et al.*'s paper reports the results of an evaluation of half-day interdisciplinary workshops, in which students share information about their programme of study, hear a carer's story and explore how team-working had an impact on the care provided. Results of the workshops have been positive and this would indeed seem to be a worthwhile activity that could be developed around palliative care for children. While many positive effects of IPE are reported in the literature, methodologically sound studies are lacking (Sloper 2004). Furthermore, the authors are unaware of any studies relating to the effectiveness of IPE within palliative care for children. Clearly, there is much scope for the development of this area from an educational perspective.

McNeilly and Price (2007) provide guidance in relation to improving the performance of the paediatric palliative care team. A central component of this guidance is the need to put the child and family first, and this should be uppermost in the minds of those involved. We have already said that health care professionals have a lack of understanding around each others' roles and do not actively communicate about the goals of care for their patients. Therefore, the first step in improving the performance of the children's palliative care team concerns the formation of achievable goals, aims and objectives for the whole team. While individuals will no doubt be familiar with these, it is important to devise these collectively across disciplines and agencies, and to revisit them on a regular basis to ensure that all involved share the same views. Each member's role, in relation to meeting the goals, should then be clearly delineated and agreed. If the performance of the team is being discussed specifically in relation to the care management of a particular child, the child (where appropriate) and parents should also be in agreement. Second, there must be an appropriate level of communication with the child and family in order to maintain a therapeutic, supportive relationship in which families can talk candidly with all members of the team. Good interpersonal communication skills are of the utmost importance here, and communication should be sufficient to avoid duplication of tasks and avoid the risk of conflicting information caused by too many people being involved. Appropriate leadership and facilitative systems should be in place to ensure the passage of information between professionals as appropriate. The identification of a key worker, in discussion with the child and family, is an integral part of this. Also related to communication is the increasing use of information technology as a means of communication, not least within the realm of e-records, the benefits and difficulties of which are currently being debated.

Third, there is a great need for co-operation within the team (McNeilly and Price, 2007). The development of mutual trust and respect is paramount if team members are to support each other (and in so doing, the child and family) in difficult circumstances, for example in the period up to and after the death of a child. Team members bring together a wide variety of skills and knowledge, and drawing on the experience of others is a vital tool within the palliative care setting. As always, children and their parents should be involved in decision-making, as it is they who know their child best.

Finally, and perhaps most important, is the need for the team to be dynamic (McNeilly and Price 2007), committed and have a positive outlook, especially given the challenges of working within the health care agenda, which is continuously changing and adapting to the needs of patients, and even more so in the case of children requiring a palliative approach to care. The performance of the team should be revisited regularly and reflected upon by all members from all agencies, either during team meetings or case conferences, or more formally during team-building exercises. Inter-agency team-building or away days are a rare event, but these could produce real differences in the functioning of the team in addition to boosting morale on both a group and an individual basis. It is generally accepted in the business world that investing in team-building initiatives is money well spent, though research within palliative care has shown that it needs to be done on an ongoing basis, as one might expect. In a study by Donaghy and Devlin (2002), while team-building in a palliative care setting had a positive effect on team-working and relationships within the team, some aspects of the improvement wore off after six months (Donaghy and Devlin 2002). Clearly, regular and timely team-building is essential if it is to be effective. An integral part of this should involve team assessment in that the team performance cannot be improved without some sort of baseline measurement of how the team is performing. While the mechanisms of team assessment are beyond the scope of this chapter, interested readers are referred to Payne (2000, ch.3) Similarly, in relation to specific team-building activities that are particularly suited to this area of practice, readers are referred to Malcolm Payne's chapter in Speck (2006), and to Benson and Rice (2007). The latter is a Royal College of Nursing Publication that recommends simple, practical team-building exercises for health care teams.

================================ **ACTIVITY** ================================

On the basis of the previous section, consider how the performance of your own team could be enhanced.

Conclusion

The needs of the child with a life-limiting or terminal illness and their wider family cannot be met by one professional alone. This chapter has demonstrated the need for both statutory and voluntary health, social care and educational services to work together across the primary, secondary and tertiary interface. Improving such co-ordination between services and agencies is key to improving outcomes for these children and their families (RCPCH 2006). However, this is particularly challenging as commitment and the need for change needs to be embraced on an individual, organizational and multi-organizational level (Sloper 2004). Individual team member have different attributes, skills and knowledge, and we need to capitalize on these so that the sum of the team's effort is greater than the parts, and the ultimate goals of care can be achieved. Stress on paediatric palliative care teams is great, therefore it makes sense that successful team-working should result in teams that feel less stressed and are therefore less prone to burnout. As a result, communication, support mechanisms within the team and outcomes for patients, in this case children and families, should also be enhanced (Firth-Cozens 2001).

Clearly, there is a great need for investment in teams providing palliative care for children, in terms of money and time, if services are to be improved. There is also a great need for research within this area of practice: for example, in relation to parents' and children's views; current practice as perceived by health care professionals; and the incidence and effectiveness of specific team assessment and team-building activities.

Key resources

ACT (Association for Children with life-threatening or terminal conditions and their families) (2004) *A Framework for the Development of Integrated Multi-Agency Care Pathways for Children with Life-Threatening and Life-Limiting Conditions*. Bristol: ACT.

Payne, M. (2000) *Teamwork in Multiprofessional Care*. Basingstoke: Palgrave.

Speck, P. (2006) *Teamwork in Palliative Care. Fulfilling or Frustrating?* Oxford: Oxford University Press.

CHAPTER SUMMARY

- The needs of the child with life-limiting or terminal illness and their wider family cannot be met by one professional alone.

- Children and parents are valued and pivotal members of the team.

- Successful teamwork is a fundamental part of caring for children with palliative care needs.

- The paediatric palliative care team is unique in terms of size and diversity and this can have an impact on the care negotiated with the child and family.

- A key to future development within this area is the need for individuals to gain further insight into the roles of others who care for children requiring palliative care. Inter-professional education in paediatric palliative care may facilitate this process.

- Individuals need to be taught how to operate within a team, and how to deal with problems as they arise. A reflective ethos can assist this process. Interdisciplinary/interagency team assessment and team- building are essential.

- Interdisciplinary working is not without its challenges, and more research needs to be done in this area if this aspect of service provision is to be improved.

References

Abbott, D., Townsley, R. and Watson, D. (2005) Multi-agency working in services for disabled children: what impact does it have on professionals? *Health and Social Care in the Community* **13**: 155–63.

ACT (Association for Children with Life-Threatening or Terminal Conditions and their Families) (2003) *Assessment of Children with Life-Limiting Conditions and Their Families. A Guide to Effective Care Planning*. Bristol: ACT.

ACT (Association for Children with Life-Threatening or Terminal Conditions and their Families (2004) *A Framework for the Development of Integrated Multi-Agency Care Pathways for Children with Life-Threatening and Life-Limiting Conditions*. Bristol: ACT.

Barton, L. and Clarke, L. (2005) *Altogether Now. An Evaluation of the Key Working Process in Warwickshire: First Report*. Stoneleigh: Integrated Disability Service.

Benson, A. and Rice, M. (eds) (2007) *Developing and Sustaining Effective Teams*. London: RCN.

Bliss, J., Cowley, S. and While, A. (2000) Interprofessional working in palliative care in the community: a review of the literature. *Journal of Interprofessional Care* **14**(3): 281–90.

Cott, C. (1998) Structure and meaning in multidisciplinary teamwork. *Sociology of Health and Illness.* **20**(6): 848–73.

Court Report, The (1976) *Fit for the Future: Report of the Committee on Child Health Services.* London: HMSO.

Craft, A. and Killen, S. (2007) *Palliative Care Services for Children and Young People in England.* Available at: www.dh.gov.uk/en/Publicationsandstatistics/Publications/PublicationsPolicyandGuidance/ DH_074459.

Crawford, G. B. and Price, S. D. (2003) Team working: palliative care as a model of interdisciplinary practice. *The Medical Journal of Australia* **179**(6 Supplement): S32-S34.

Davies, R. (2006) The potential of integrated multi-agency care pathways for children. *British Journal of Nursing* **15**(14): 764–8.

DfES (Department for Education and Skills) (2005) Common Core Skills for the Children's Workforce. Available at: wwweverychildmatters.gov.uk/deliveryservices/commoncore/multi agencyworking; Accessed 13 August 2007.

DfES and DH (Department for Education and Skills and Department of Health (2004a) *National Service Framework for Children, Young People and Maternity Services. Disabled Children and Young People and Those with Complex Health Needs* Available at: www.dh.gov.uk/en/PublicationsandStatistics/ Publications/PublicationsPolicyAndGuidance/DH_4089112

DfES and DH (Department for Education and Skills and Department of Health (2004b) *Early Support: Professional Guidance.* Nottingham: DfES Publications.

DH (Department of Health) (2006) *Our Health, Our* Care, Our *Say: A New Direction for Community Services.* Available at: www.dh.gov.uk/en/Publicationsandstatistics/Publications/Publications PolicyandGuidance/DH_4127453; accessed 14 August 2007.

DH (Department of Health) (2008) *Better Care: Better Lives. Improving Outcomes and Experiences for Children, Young People and Their Families Living with Life-Limiting and Life-Threatening Conditions.* London: Department of Health.

Donaghy, K. and Devlin, B. (2002) An evaluation of teamwork within a specialist palliative care unit. *International Journal of Palliative Nursing* **8**(11): 518–25.

Drinka, T. J. K. and Clark, P. G. (2000) *Health Care Teamwork. Interdisciplinary Practice and Teaching.* London: Auburn House.

Firth-Cozens, J. (2001) Multidisciplinary teamwork: the good, bad and everything in between. *Quality in Health Care* **10**: 65–9.

General Medical Council (2003) *Tomorrow's Doctors.* Available at: www.gmc-uk.org/education/ undergraduate_policy/tomorrows_doctors.asp; accessed 29 September 2007.

Greco, V. and Sloper, P. (2004) Care co-ordination and key worker schemes for disabled children: results of a UK-wide survey. *Child: Care, Health and Development* **30**: 13–20.

Greco, V., Sloper, P., Webb, R. and Beecham, J. (2005) *An Exploration of Different Models of Multiagency Partnerships in Key Worker Services for Disabled Children: Effectiveness and Costs.* Nottingham: DfES.

Greco, V., Sloper, P., Webb, R. and Beecham, J. (2007) Key worker services for disabled children: the views of parents. *Children and Society* **21**(3): 162–74.

Hawryluck, L. and Ryan, D. (2001) *Ian Anderson Continuing Education Program in End-of-life Care. Collaboration.* Available at: www.cme.utoronto.ca/EndOfLife/Modules/COLLABORATION%20 MODULE.pdf; accessed 22 October 2008.

Headrick, L. A., Wilcock, P. M. and Batalden, P. B. (1998) Interprofessional working and continuing medical education. *British Medical Journal* **316**: 771–4.

Hill, A. (1998) Multiprofessional teamwork in hospital palliative care teams. *International Journal of Palliative Nursing* **4**(5): 214–21.

Jack, B., Hillier, V., Williams, A., and Oldham, J. (2004) Hospital based palliative care teams improve the insight of cancer patients into their disease. *Palliative Medicine* **18**: 46–52.

Jassal, S. S. and Sims, J. Working as a team. In Goldman, A., Hain, R. and Liben, S. (eds) (2006) *Oxford Textbook of Palliative Care for Children*. Oxford University Press.

Kirk, S. and Glendinning, C. (2004) Developing services to support parents caring for a technology dependent child at home. *Child: Care, Health and Development* **30**(3): 209–18.

Limbrick, P. (2004) *Early Support for Children with Complex Needs. Team Around the Child and the Multi-Agency Key Worker.* Hereford: Interconnections.

Limbrick, P. (2005) Principles and practices that define the Team-Around-the-Child (TAC) approach and their relationship to accepted good practice (Working paper). Hereford: Interconnections.

Luthans, F. (2002) *Organisational Behaviour* (9th edn). New York: McGraw-Hill.

McNeilly, P. and Price, J. (2007) Interdisciplinary teamworking in paediatric palliative care. *European Journal of Palliative Care* **14**(2): 64–7.

Myers, D. (2008) *Social Psychology* (9th edn). New York: McGraw-Hill.

Nursing and Midwifery Council (2004) *Standards of Proficiency for Pre-registration Education*. London: NMC.

O'Connor, M., Fisher, C. and Guilfoyle, A. (2006) Interdisciplinary teams in palliative care: a critical reflection. *International Journal of Palliative Nursing* **12**(3): 132–7.

Partridge, L. (2007) *Teams. Learning Made Simple*. London: Elsevier.

Payne, M. (2000) Teamwork in Multiprofessional Care. Basingstoke: Palgrave.

Price, J. and McNeilly, P. (2006) Developing an educational programme in paediatric palliative care. *International Journal of Palliative Nursing* **2**(11): 536–41.

Pritchard, P. and Pritchard, J. (1994) *Teamwork for Primary and Shared Care: A Practical Workbook.* Oxford: Oxford University Press.

RCPCH (Royal College of Paediatrics and Child Health) (2006) *A Guide to Understanding Pathways and Implementing Networks*. London: RCPCH.

Rushmer, R. (2005) Blurred boundaries damage inter-professional working. *Nurse Researcher* **12**(3): 74–85.

Schrader, S. L., Horner, A., Eidsness, L., Young, S., Wright, C. and Robinson, M. (2002) A team approach in palliative care: Enhancing outcomes. *South Dakota Journal of Medicine* **55**(7): 269–78.

Sealey, P. and Feuer, D. (2007) How do hospital palliative care teams liaise with their colleagues? *European Journal of Palliative Care* **14**(2): 75–7.

Sloper, P. (2004) Facilitators and barriers for co-ordinated multi-agency services. *Child: Care, Health and Development* **30**(6): 571–80.

Sloper, P., Greco, V., Beecham, J. and Webb, R. (2005) Key worker services for disabled children: what characteristics of services lead to better outcomes for children and families? *Child: Care, Health and Development* **32**(2): 147–57.

Speck, P. (2006) *Teamwork in Palliative Care. Fulfilling or Frustrating?* Oxford: Oxford University Press.

Steele, R. G. (2002) Experiences of families in which a child has a prolonged terminal illness: modifying factors. *International Journal of Palliative Nursing* **8**(9): 418–34.

Townsley, R. Abbott, D. and Watson, D. (2004) *Making a Difference: Exploring the Impact of Multi-agency Working on Disabled Children with Complex Care Needs, Their Families and the Professionals Who Support Them.* Bristol: Policy Press.

Tuckman, R. W. (1965) Developmental sequence in small groups. *Psychological Bulletin* **63**(6): 384–99.

Warr, B. (2007) Working collaboratively. In Brown, E. *Supporting the Child and the Family in Paediatric Palliative Care*. London: Jessica Kingsley.

Watson, D., Townsley, R. and Abbott, D. (2002) Exploring multi-agency working in services to disabled children with complex healthcare needs and their families. *Journal of Clinical Nursing* **11**: 367–75.

Wee, B., Hillier, R., Coles, C., Mountford, B., Sheldon, F. and Turner, P. (2001) Palliative care: a suitable setting for undergraduate interprofessional education. *Palliative Medicine* **15**: 487–92.

3

Communicating Effectively

Jayne Price and Carole Cairns

Introduction

Good levels of concise, skilled and effective communication are recognized as fundamental within the area of children's palliative care (ACT 2003). The facilitation and documentation of communication has been described as one of the basic principles of palliative care for children (Kane *et al.* 2004) and as such is pivotal within the interdisciplinary team approach to caring for children and families. Communicating information to children and families about illness and care ensures they are empowered with the knowledge required to make informed decisions, which is undoubtedly a central component to partnership working (McNeilly *et al.* 2006). It is for these reasons that Foster (2007) affirms that effective communication is a critical attribute in children's palliative care.

Despite the recognition of the centrality of good communication, the interplay between the complex sociological and psychological issues surrounding the child and their family can make the process extremely challenging. Evidence from families endorses the belief that communication with staff can be unsatisfactory (Davies and Connaughty 2002) and result in confusion and distress (Contro *et al.* 2004).

Given that good communication and quality of care are inextricably linked, issues around communication were a strand running through the preceding chapters, and will continue to be in the remaining chapters of this book. This chapter aims to deepen understanding of the concepts and strategies that can assist the interdisciplinary team in overcoming communication challenges experienced when caring for children and families throughout the different stages of the palliative care 'journey'.

> ## KEY POINT
>
> An effective level of communication is essential at each stage of the palliative care journey.

Definitions of communication

Peel (2003) identifies that the process of communicating information involves a sender, a medium, a message and the recipient, while Bradley and Edinberg (1982) asserted that communication is a process by which information is transmitted through verbal and non-verbal means. Brooks and Heath (1985) also include the exchange of meanings and feelings in their explanation of what constitutes communication. Within health care, trust and honesty are viewed as essential components in the two-way process between patient and health care professional (Cooley 2000) and are key to a therapeutic relationship. It is important that health and social care professionals recognize that information provided may not necessarily be understood fully or retained by the receiver (van der Molen 2007).

This chapter is therefore based on the premise that communication within children's palliative care is a process where information and messages are shared between individuals and groups through verbal and non-verbal methods in a culture that fosters trust, honesty and respect.

Communication context in children's palliative care

As caring for children with palliative care needs and their families evokes many emotional issues, and reactions, the need to communicate compassionately with the child and family cannot be understated. Time and consideration are essential (WMPMT 2005), alongside therapeutic communication skills such as supporting, observing, interviewing and listening, all of which have been identified as valuable when working with families (Steele 2002).

Moreover, guiding the family and child (if appropriate) through options requires self-awareness, emotional maturity, sensitivity and empathy (Kuttner 2007). The ability of staff to communicate sensitively and effectively at the end of a child's life was investigated in a study that collected data from forty-five bereaved parents whose children had died in hospital (Davies and Connaughty 2002). Only a fifth (n = 9) of the parents were satisfied with the staff's ability to communicate. The perceptions of parents indicated that the staff appeared so focused on cure and treatment they found it difficult to communicate adequately with parents whose child was not curable. The parents in this study clearly recommended that interactions should be on a person to person basis rather than professional to parent, and furthermore indicated that being 'professional' should not over shadow basic human concern and caring.

Families themselves identify the link between inadequate and ineffective communication and increased confusion and /or distress. Insensitive comments by professionals caused families much pain and complicated their grief reaction (Contro *et al.* 2004).

Legislation also endorses the importance of effective communication with children, young people and families within the field of palliative care. The ACT Charter (2004a), IMPaCCT (2007) and the ICPCN Charter (2008) corroborate that information should be provided for the parent, the child, siblings and other relatives, appropriate to their age and understanding. This diversity is one of the reasons why communication within the field of children's palliative care can be difficult.

Barriers to communication

Barriers to effective communication exist throughout the different stages of the child's and family's journey. These barriers can be environmental; for example, a busy, noisy ward can have multiple distractions and there may also be a lack of privacy. The environment within the child's home – for example, the television, other family members or noisy pets – can hinder good communication (Cooley 2005). Physical and emotional barriers between individuals or groups can also have an impact on the quality of interaction.

ACTIVITY

Read the Clinical Focus scenario below and consider the barriers to communication inherent in this. What factors could have a negative influence on the quality of the communication between the child's family and the nurse?

CLINICAL FOCUS

Mohammed is a 7-year-old boy with an undiagnosed genetic condition. He has severe development delay and frequent seizure activity. He has limited movement and is wheelchair dependent. His nutritional intake is maintained by enteral feeding via a low profile gastrostomy device. The interdisciplinary team consist of professionals from health, education, social work and voluntary services.

The family have lived with the constant threat of death and uncertainty over the years, and there have been a few periods where he was very ill and death was the expected outcome on those occasions. Despite this, he survived. He has deteriorated considerably in the last few months and is ill with another chest infection. Mum is certain that this latest infection will be like all the others and that he will recover. He is the youngest of five children and lives at home with his parents and paternal grandmother. Mum is the main carer and speaks limited English. Dad speaks Urdu and English fluently.

The Community Children's Nursing team (CCN team) has been involved with Mohammed's care with differing levels of input over the last six years. Recently, the CCN who was their key worker has moved to another post and a new key worker, also a CCN, has been appointed.

The CCN team work closely with an Urdu interpreter in caring for Mohammed. A skilled and experienced interpreter is essential to ensure that Mohammed and his family receive appropriate care. It has not always been possible to book an interpreter, and maintaining continuity is also difficult as the same interpreter was not always available. When the interpreter is not available, the team interpreted through other family members. However, this was difficult as these family members do not have the skills of a trained interpreter, which also raises issues of confidentiality.

Dad has openly expressed that he feels his son is dying and the child's grandmother appears hostile to the CCN, believing that some curative treatment should be available for Mohammed. When the CCN visits Mohammed and his family there are always large numbers of extended family in the home.

INTERDISCIPLINARY INSIGHT

The role of the CCN in ensuring effective communication when caring for Mohammed and his family

- To provide effective communication at all levels, both with the family and between inter-disciplinary team.
- To liaise with all members of the interdisciplinary team; for example, the React Nurse, Interpreter, District Nurse, GP, Hospital Consultant, Pain Team.
- To listen to and enable the family (both Mum and Dad) while forming a therapeutic relationship.
- To help the family communicate fears, anxieties and anger as appropriate.
- To provide comprehensive information for the family (including siblings and extended family) that is easily understood.
- To ensure the care package meets the needs of the child and family, addressing cultural influences and needs.
- To direct family to appropriate sources of information and help.
- To communicate with the child by appropriate means; for example, non-verbal.
- To co-ordinate service provision in the role of a key worker.
- To liaise with key people/act as an access point to other services.
- To continually evaluate the family's understanding of information given.
- To help the family to identify and build on existing coping mechanisms.
- To assess the child/family's needs on an ongoing basis.
- To help the family solve problems.
- To provide emotional support for the child and family.
- To enable the family to maintain control of the situation.
- To teach the family to carry out specific nursing care.
- To empower the parents to feel competent and confident when caring for their child.
- To teach/educate other members of the interdisciplinary team.
- To act as an advocate for the child and family.

Written by Elizabeth Gillespie, Community Children's Nurse.

The scenario on page 41 illustrates some of the many factors that can influence the quality of interaction between a child, the family and health care professionals.

Undoubtedly, emotions have an important role to play within the communication process. Knowing a child has a limited life span causes a family anxiety, fear, distress and sadness, and this has a clear correlation with what an individual may be willing or able to interpret or understand. Fear too can impinge on the way health and social care professionals communicate; for example, concern about what to say to families, and fear of saying the wrong thing.

The family may feel angry that treatment/technology has failed their child, or not be willing to accept that their child may die. Constant media bombardment with medical 'breakthroughs' leads to high expectations of 'miracle' cures. This ensuing anger and denial may hinder effective communication as well as decision-making and care delivery. Families may also find it difficult to accept the reality of death, especially if previous predictions have proved inaccurate or the child improved at a time when death was expected (AAP 2000). Individuals react in different ways, and each member of the interdisciplinary team must be aware of this.

A good working relationship with parents alongside the development of a rapport with children and families to enable the demonstration of understanding, respect and honesty is essential. Anything that can have a negative impact on the therapeutic relationship can therefore present as a barrier to care provision and communication. For example, many parents may have cared for their children over a number of years with increasing medical needs and dependency, therefore developing expertise. Hewitt–Taylor (2005) identify that working with 'expert parents' can be particularly daunting for members of the interdisciplinary team, which may create tensions within the therapeutic relationship. Families also report the importance of continuity, and a health care professional who is familiar to them and their child (Contro *et al.* 2004); this may be difficult to maintain and indicates that families may not be as open with a professional who does not know them or their child well.

Cooley (2000) concedes that recognizing individuality will enable the health and social care professional to realize that essential skills in the art of communication include listening, intuition and sensitivity. Language and cultural influences too can be a barrier to effective communication when working with families (WMPMT 2005) and require careful consideration, as in the clinical focus scenario on page 40.

Age and cognitive ability of the child is another influential factor when considering communication. Parents of children with complex health needs have highlighted that their child's difficulty in speaking was often mistaken for a lack of understanding (Hewitt–Taylor 2008). Non-verbal communication techniques are therefore important strategies, particularly with young children or children with specific communication difficulties (Downs and Simons, 2006); these include body language, facial expression, eyebrows, hands and noises (Hewitt–Taylor 2008).

While barriers to effective communication exist, these they are not insurmountable. The clinical scenario illustrates how barriers could be overcome with careful consideration, negotiation and understanding from the CCN and interdisciplinary team in each aspect of care throughout the child's journey.

Specific communication challenges within children's palliative care

Complex and challenging communication issues can arise, with the communication needs of a child and family changing over time. Assessment must therefore be carried out on an ongoing basis by the interdisciplinary team providing the care.

Receiving the diagnosis or bad news, negotiating contradictions and confusion, getting the correct amount of information, the importance of good communication and feeling listened to were raised as communication issues by parents who had a child diagnosed with cancer (Clarke and Fletcher 2003).

Staff too report difficulty in this aspect of care provision. A study by Contro *et al.* (2004) reported that staff felt inexperienced in four specific areas of communication with children and families. These were: the transition from curative to palliative care, discussing end-of-life issues with families, discussion of end- of- life issues with children and discussion around do-not-resuscitate (DNR) status. Education, training and support, as well as clinical supervision and reflection may help staff to overcome feelings of inadequacy in these areas and assist in developing good practice. Staff who are well supported and confident in their practice are more likely to convey this to those in their care (WMPMT 2005).

Examples of some of the challenges are summarized in Figure 3.1, you may identify others. It is essential to remember that these challenges will differ, depending on the individual child and family's particular situation and circumstances.

As conflict within teams has been explored in Chapter 2, this will not be repeated here. Decision-making, decisions around withdrawal of treatment and DNR orders will be discussed in depth in Chapter 4 of the book, and while there is some overlap, these will not be explored extensively here. The intricacies of communicating with bereaved families is the subject of Chapter 10. Therefore, the remainder of this chapter will examine the first four of these challenges and outline relevant concepts and strategies that can assist health and social care professionals to communicate effectively in practice.

- Breaking bad news
- Sharing information
- Discussing death with children and families
- Negotiating conflicts
- Decisions around withdrawing treatment and DNR
- Decision-making
- Conflict within teams
- Communication with bereaved families

Figure 3.1 Examples of communication challenges in children's palliative care

Breaking bad news

> Every family should receive the disclosure of their child's prognosis in a face-to-face discussion in privacy and should be treated with respect, honesty and sensitivity (ACT 2004b: 16).

Breaking bad news has been considered one of the most complex and challenging communication encounters within children's palliative care (Price *et al.* 2006). Given that 'breaking bad news' means imparting information that will drastically change a person's future life for the worse (Buckman 1992, Kaye 1996) then telling parents of their child's life-limiting/life-threatening diagnosis, relapse or impending death must be the epitome of bad news (ACT 2004b).

═══════════════════ **ACTIVITY** ═══════════════════

Consider the types of bad news that might be broken to parents within children's palliative care. From your experience in practice, consider the factors that may influence a parent's ability to receive bad news.

Receiving the news that their child has an illness or disability that will place restrictions on any aspect of family life, or that the child has a life-limiting or life-threatening illness, is extremely difficult for parents (Matthews 2006). The manner in which the bad news is broken can influence the ability of the child/family to cope, and potentially their relationship with the health care team (Contro *et al.* 2002). In the case of communicating a serious diagnosis, it is from this point that parents should understand that they are entering a partnership in caring for their child (ACT 2004b).

Twycross (2003: 25) asserts that 'when and how to tell' is central to the process of breaking bad news. The importance of good communication skills when breaking bad news to parents must not be understated, and parents report the

---

- Preparation.
- Establish what the parent knows.
- Is more information required by the parents?
- Give a warning.
- Permit parental denial.
- Explain in easily understood terms.
- Listen to parental concerns.
- Encourage parental feelings to be expressed.
- Summarize, check understanding and make a plan.
- Offer continual support and availability.

Figure 3.2 A 10-step approach to breaking bad news to parents

Source: Adapted from Kaye (1996).

importance of hearing difficult news from a familiar health care professional who communicates with them in a clear, honest and compassionate manner (Contro *et al.* 2004). If the manner adopted is abrupt, this can be remembered even when the initial shock has passed, and will form a poor basis for future communication. Effectively communicating bad news therefore is not an optional skill but should be considered an obligatory part of a professional's practice (DHSSPS 2003).

Many respected authors have written extensively about the skills required to break bad news (Buckman 1992, Kaye 1996), and guidelines have been produced (Kaye 1996, Baile *et al.* 2000, DHSSPS 2003).

Frameworks can guide professionals in breaking bad news; however, their use must incorporate flexibility whilst recognizing the uniqueness of each family and situation. Breaking bad news should be carefully planned, clearly presented and delivered with compassion (Price *et al.* 2006).

Within children's palliative care, the breaking of bad news is normally the role of the child's consultant. The named nurse/key worker or social worker may also be present. The initial meeting is usually with the parents, though some older children and young people may be involved in this consultation. Whether the child or young person is present is dependent on the individual child, or young person and his or her family.

The case study below illustrates such a consultation with a family and outlines the role of the doctor in this process.

CLINICAL FOCUS

Jenny is a 5-year-old girl who was admitted to a district hospital with abdominal distension. Radiology suggests abdominal neuroblastoma. She is referred to the Regional Oncology Unit for further investigation.

The Consultant and Jenny's named nurse are to meet with the parents in the ward office while Jenny stays with the Play Specialist on the ward. Speaking to parents on their own initially gives the doctor and parents the opportunity to interact without any distractions, and gives parents the chance to assimilate the information and express their emotions without this being witnessed by the child. Following introductions, the parents settle on two chairs together, while the consultant sits adjacent to them, with the nurse on the other side.

Trying to establish what the parents know, the consultant asks what the doctor in the other hospital told them. Mum denies being given any information. Dad was not there and is quite agitated that his wife was 'left in the dark'. To gently find out exactly what they know, the consultant asks them to tell Jenny's story. Mum talks hesitantly but continues as she admits the other doctor said something about a 'lump in her tummy'. The consultant maintains eye contact and encourages her with nods, repeating some of her words when she falters. Dad sits forward, pointing his finger repeatedly in the air, demanding that the lump must be removed immediately, and mentions his mother. The consultant asks what he means by this, and both parents start to cry. Eventually Dad says his mother had a 'tumour'.

While the nurse offers tissues, they sit in silence then the consultant asks whether or not the parents want to continue at this stage. Dad looks at Mum and when she nods he asks the consultant to continue.

He warns that the ultrasound does show that Jenny has a lump in her tummy and expresses concern. Jenny's parents are silent, but hold hands. The consultant then expresses their concern that Jenny has a tumour. After probing their understanding, he explains gently that the tumour is probably a cancer.

Mum appears to start to talk and then stops.

Giving the parents an opportunity to express their feelings, the consultant asks them their thoughts on this. Dad shares that with Jenny's Granny, nothing could be done.

The consultant explains that childhood cancers are very different from adult cancers and assures them that when all the test results are back they will able to be discuss Jenny's treatment. Mum then turns and stares out of the window. Dad asks about the proposed scan. A plan is given for blood tests that afternoon and a CT can in the morning.

Before leaving the room, the consultant arranges to meet with them at 2pm the next day with the results and to discuss the way forward he also offers his regret at having to tell them such news. The nurse remains with the parents to offer further support and they express their concern about how they would explain the situation to their daughter. The nurse guides and supports them in this matter.

INTERDISCIPLINARY INSIGHT

The role of the doctor in breaking bad news incorporating Kaye (1996)

Preparation
- Be familiar with history and test results
- Know immediate management options
- Anticipate questions
- Liaise with named nurse

Support
- Ensure supportive professionals during and after consultation
- Both parents together if possible
- Ensure privacy of setting
- Be aware of body language indicating interest and empathy
- Provide tissues

Sharing information
- Find out what the parents know
- Find out what the parents want to know
- Warning shots
- Give the 'news' in sections and establish understanding – 'chunk 'n' check'
- Avoid medical jargon
- Ask concerns and listen verbal/non-verbal: summarize, encouraging words, repetition, empathic response, touch, silences, body language, eye contact
- Written information to back up verbal
- Allow initial denial

Venting emotions
- Ask open questions
- Listen – empathetic; therapeutic
- Allow silences

Maintain hope
- Avoid unrealistic promises
- Realistic goals
- Acknowledge uncertainties but offer review

Follow-up
- Implies future support
- Allows discussion of detail on repeat explanation
- Allows time for organization of family support
- Allows emotional adjustment

Afterwards
- Reflection on feeling and facts for all parties
- Communication: written notes, records for all professionals involved, record for future consultations
- Professional to professional:
- hospital/ community,
- key workers,
- interdisciplinary team meetings

FURTHER READING

Read the article by Price *et al.* (2006) and consider the role of the children's nurse in offering support to families.

Breaking bad news will give rise to strong feelings among both family and/or the professionals involved. In the case of Jenny's family, gendered differences in parental reactions are apparent (Steele 2002, Downs and Simons 2006). Parents can experience a myriad of emotions and the reaction is similar to a grief reaction, where a degree of anticipatory grief can be experienced (Dighe *et al.* 2008). This is discussed in Chapter 10.

The Kübler-Ross (1970) stages of dying are useful when considering how families, or indeed the children themselves, may react to hearing the news of a serious diagnosis or a poor prognosis (see Figure 3.3).

In addition to the emotions identified by Kübler-Ross (1970) feelings of fear, helplessness, hopelessness and isolation can also be experienced. On being

- Denial
- Anger
- Bargaining
- Depression
- Acceptance

Figure 3.3 Stages of dying

Source: Kübler-Ross (1970).

presented with bad news regarding their child's future, parents may feel judged that they have failed the child (Downs and Simons 2006) or guilt in the case of genetic conditions; these feelings may conspire to affect their coping.

Breaking bad news implies giving the truth, but in a sensitive and caring manner (Mack *et al.* 2005). To achieve the effective breaking of bad news: that is, to initiate the course of future care, then information, including views, expectations and emotions, must be elicited from the parents. Listening to parents and hearing their concerns are two of the most important skills for communication in palliative care (Cooley 2005). Showing empathy, speaking the truth and expressing sadness to the family are also salient (Kuttner 2007).

The capacity of some parents to make a rational decision can be compromised by their emotions (Larcher 2006); therefore, the professional has a duty to give a balanced presentation of benefits/disadvantages and enough time to reflect on these (RCPCH 2004, GMC 2006). Though the child remains at the centre of the interdisciplinary team's ethical and legal duty, there is a moral duty to the parents in the area of guidance, and in relief of their distress (Larcher 2006).

Parents have a need for information at this time (Starke and Mollers 2002, ACT 2004b). Information should be provided for the child (as appropriate) and family in language that is easily understood. Interpreters should be used if necessary. Written information to back up that given verbally is also important (Price *et al.* 2006). Information in addition to the maintenance of open channels of communication between the interdisciplinary team, child and family provide the necessary platform for decision-making (Anghelescu *et al.* 2006).

For the professional, the task of giving bad news, or being present when bad news is given, can give rise to reactions similar to those experienced by those receiving the news (Hindmarch 2000). Acknowledging that treatment is not available for a child, or that a child is approaching death, may render the professional open to guilt that they in some way have failed the child and the family (Costello and Trinder-Brook 2000). Emotions can emerge from previous experiences, both personal and professional. Recognizing one's own reactions and emotions can reduce their effect on future communications and prevent a judgemental attitude (ways of supporting staff are discussed in Chapter 9).

Communicating bad news to families is a frequent and vitally important aspect of care provision within children's palliative care, yet the need for more education in this area has been identified (Kolarik *et al.* 2006).

Sharing information

Sharing information is recognized as being essential for partnership working between children, their families and the different members of the interdisciplinary team (Hummelinck and Pollock 2006, Thurgate 2006). Sharing information within the caring context is a two-way process, and the interdisciplinary team must be receptive to information and insights offered by parents (WMPMT 2005). Respecting and listening to information given by parents regarding their child can aid them in feeling in control, while not listening can invoke frustration and anger (Clarke and Fletcher 2003). Parents can give invaluable insights into key events such as the development of new symptoms, and what works for their child (WMPMT 2005).

Honest and complete information in an understandable form has also been identified as being important to families (Steele 2002, Meyer *et al.* 2006). Information should be given in a clear and concise manner (Price 2003) and the need to reiterate information to families and constantly assess their level of understanding is essential (WMPMT 2005). An awareness that parental need for information changes over time is important (Patterson Kelly and Porock 2005). Furthermore, James and Johnson (1997) reported that parents have an increased need for information as their child approaches the end of life.

KEY POINT

Information is essential to ensure that families are empowered with the knowledge to make decisions about their child's care.

In a world that is increasingly technology-driven, the amount of information available has multiplied, with the internet offering a viable medium for parents to access information (Blackburn and Read 2005). While the members of the interdisciplinary team will provide the principal information, it is not unusual for parents, and indeed children, to seek additional information from other sources. Information from the internet is often used to influence parents' decisions regarding their child's care (Wainstein *et al.* 2006). It is suggested that enabling patients to procure information via several media may improve patient–doctor communication (Coulter *et al.* 1999). It has also been suggested that incorporating patient-researched information should be seen as an additional element of that professional relationship (Stark 2003).

WEB LINKS

Select a condition affecting a child/children you have looked after. Search the internet, noting the number and quality of some internet resources available for families about your chosen condition.

While the type of information accessible via the internet can be positive (Price 2003), sometimes the quality of the information is poor, and families can become confused when faced with inaccurate or conflicting information (Wainstein *et al.* 2006). Parents also may find multiple 'miracle cures' on the internet. This may be the coping reaction of denial and needs to be dealt with gently. This can induce many emotions and concerns within the professional: defensiveness, uncertainty, and ethical worry on behalf of the child's best interests or the family's financial risk. The interdisciplinary team must work with families to help them understand, evaluate and prioritize the information they receive and discover (ACT 2004b).

Given that a family-centred approach is fundamental in the delivery of palliative care to children, families must be welcomed into the care arena and empowered with suitable knowledge and the information required to be actively involved in both care and the decision-making process. Palliative care for children is made even more complex by the fact that children are unable to act autonomously in the decision-making process; the parents are usually nominated as surrogate decision-makers (Hynson *et al.* 2003).

A young person will have specific information needs similar to their parents, but care should be taken to recognize the individual's level of understanding and family relationships (Young *et al.* 2003). They are at a stage of wanting privacy and autonomy, and resent dependence on adults (both family and professionals) because of physical illness. Young people can provide mutual support and this should be encouraged by providing meeting facilities, either during treatments or socially (Thornes 2001).

Children too require information. The nature of the tripartite relationship means that the child is central and requires the same information as the family (Price and McFarlane 2006). It is vitally important to consider the specific needs of children when giving them information about their illness, treatment or care (Price 2003). These considerations are highlighted in Figure 3.4.

Some families may not want their children to know some details; for example, that death is approaching. Talking to children about illness and death is extremely difficult, and careful attention must be given to the child's developmental stage (Hynson *et al.* 2003) thus ensuring easily understood information tailored to the needs of the individual child. The interdisciplinary team members working with children require a knowledge of growth and development, and how the child's illness may in turn influence the individual child's well being (Himelstein 2006).

Story-telling (Done 2001) or other interactive methods offer choice when considering how to impart information to children (Price 2003). Play is important as it is a medium that helps children to understand their world (Hynson *et al.* 2003). As such, it has a therapeutic dimension and is an important communication tool

---

Consider the child's age and cognitive developmental stage carefully.

Highlight and establish child's current level of understanding.

Include other members of the interdisciplinary team: for example, play specialist.

Language to be used that is simple and age- appropriate.

Discuss with and involve parents.

Restrict the time of session – remember limited attention span.

Employ a range of strategies; for example, play, stories.

Necessary to establish understanding.

Figure 3.4 The specific information needs of children

Source: Price (2003). Reproduced with the kind permission of *Cancer Nursing Practice.*

for children who are ill (Price and Spence 2004). Play can be used as a way of imparting information to children, or as a means for them to express their feelings, fears and anxieties (Price and Spence 2004). The play therapist plays a key role in imparting information to children of a variety of ages (Price 2003) and in helping children express their feelings and emotions (Langton 2000).

CLINICAL FOCUS

Molly is a 6-year-old girl who has acute lymphoblastic leukaemia (ALL). She lives with her parents and 10-year-old sister, Katie. She had treatment but later relapsed and is now having her end-of-life care delivered at home. During treatment, Molly required long periods in hospital, where she built a rapport with the hospital play specialist (HPS) and the other members of the interdisciplinary team. The HPS designed an individualized play programme specific to Molly's needs, creating a normal routine in an abnormal environment. Books and stories are used to give Molly information about her illness and procedures at her own developmental level.

With no further curative treatment options available, the family wish Molly to be cared for at home. The community play specialist (CPS) is a member of the interdisciplinary team and plays a key role in end- of- life care for children at home. This will enable Molly's play programme to be adapted and continued at home as an integral part of her care package. The HPS introduces the CPS to Molly and her family. The programme will again serve as a way of promoting normality for Molly and offers a therapeutic dimension. The CPS provides a programme increasingly involving Molly's sister, parents and extended family. This is a highly sensitive package creating positive memories, providing enjoyment for Molly and in addition ensures a medium for Molly to express any anxiety or worry. The CPS works with Molly and her family to create a memory book which includes craftwork, photos and letters. Katie is supported to be involved in the play activities. Although Molly and Katie have not raised any specific issues or worries about death with the CPS, the CPS is aware through the interdisciplinary team meeting and ongoing team communication that the parents were using a selection of story-telling books recommended by the Macmillan nurse to initiate discussion about death. These resources are age-appropriate.

INTERDISCIPLINARY INSIGHT

The role of the Hospital Play Specialist (HPS) and Community Play Specialist (CPS) in Molly's palliative care

- To design an individualized play programme to meet Molly's holistic needs by reducing anxiety through familiar activities.
- All equipment used by the HPS and CPS are chosen to complement Molly's age and stage of development.
- To use play skilfully as a medium to impart information to Molly and her sister, and as a tool for the child and sibling to express their feelings and concerns.
- To observe and assess the child's anxieties, and to liaise with all members of the interdisciplinary team — both in hospital and the community-through attendance at team meetings, and to provide concise and accurate documentation.

▓ To provide sibling support and inclusion in all aspects of the child's play/palliative programme.

▓ To ensure Molly's play programme promotes continuity of care between the hospital and community.

▓ To arrange regular home visits in conjunction with the child and family (CPS).

▓ To record positive memories and events for the child and family as the end of her life approaches.

▓ To act as an advocate for the child.

▓ The palliative care package gives the whole family an opportunity to participate in a positive way with Molly.

Written by Naomi Spence and Sophie Rea.

The sharing of information among families, children and the interdisciplinary team permits integrated care and assists in the decision-making process. Accurate information that helps facilitate informed choices is essential. Decision-making should involve the child (where possible) the family and the health care professionals (Hynson *et al.* 2003).

While involving children in decision-making is widely advocated (see Chapter 4) the degree to which this is achieved in reality is unclear and is very dependant on the individual child and family (Toce 2001). Some children – for example, infants and those with severe neurological impairment – will have no capacity to participate in decisions; others will have a developing capacity; and others – for example, young people – will have the ability to make decisions (Toce 2001). Hinds *et al.* (2005) interviewed children with cancer aged over 10 years old and, within seven days of being involved in an end-of-life decision, (n = 20) 90 per cent of the children recalled with clarity all their treatment options and identified their own death as a consequence of that decision. This study demonstrates that children can have the ability and understanding to be actively involved in making choices and decisions. However, communicating with children about such issues and involving them in decisions remains contentious.

Communicating with children about death

Dilemmas exist around truth- telling and communication with children, particularly if they are approaching death. Open discussion of bad news, such as death, with children is difficult (Goldman 2007). Parents may find it easier to assume that they will not understand and not broach the subject, feeling that they want to protect their child from the truth in order to reduce fear and anxiety. However, children in the main have a deeper understanding than their parents give them credit for (Goldman 2007), and in fact by giving children the opportunity to communicate may allay their fears (Hilden *et al.* 2000). In reality, lack of knowledge and insight about what is happening to them can cause even more psychological disturbance.

■ The age and cognitive ability of the child are instrumental, and a good knowledge of this is essential when managing the care process of the child receiving palliative care.

■ The value of appreciating the existing communication system within the family.

■ The realization that effective communication can reduce anxiety.

■ The choice of the medium of communication most readily used by the child.

Figure 3.5 Key components of effective communication with children about death.

Source: Lansdown (1994).

Lansdown (1994) outlined key components of communication about death to children (see Figure 3.5) .These four principles could be central to communication with children throughout their palliative care journey and not only as they approach death, equally the health care professional could use these for talking with siblings.

Children with a life-threatening/life-limiting condition are thought to have an awareness of their own death, often sensing that their condition is serious and that they could die, even if this has not been explained to them (Judd 1998). Whether this awareness is openly acknowledged and talked about is dependant on the individual child, parents and professionals involved (Dunlop 2008)

A seminal study by Bluebond-Langer (1978) gives important insights into children's awareness about illness and death, having long established that children have an awareness of their illness and that they are dying. The study highlights that through repetitive cycles of sickness, treatment, remission and relapse, the child with a life-threatening illness moves from the perception that 'I am sick but I will get better' to 'I am sick and will eventually die from this illness.' This indicated that children go through a process of awareness of death shaped by their experience rather than their age. While the 'stages' approach is useful, this should not replace a receptiveness to the child's own cognitive ability and level of understanding, as well as their willingness to talk. Furthermore, other factors, such as cultural experiences and verbal ability, can influence an individual child's awareness (Kenyon 2001). It is also important to recognize that the child's health care experience also influences their understanding, many children will have heard of or witnessed the deterioration and death of other children with similar conditions (Dunlop 2008).

The influential work of Nagy (1948) has shaped the modern stance on children's understanding of death. The findings identified three main stages. Until the age of about five, much curiosity was common in relation to death, but there was a lack of understanding about the finality of death. Death and sleep are seen as similar concepts at this stage. During the second stage, which includes children from five to nine, the finality of death is accepted. Nagy identified that many of this age group tend to think of death as a person who takes people away. At this developmental stage, children believe death will not necessarily happen to them. From the age of 9 onwards death is viewed as inevitable, universal and final.

> ### KEY POINT
>
> Children are thought to have an awareness about illness and the fact that they are dying even if they have not been told.

Despite this apparent awareness and understanding, however, the child often remains silent in an attempt to protect his or her parents from upset, and the parent does the same to protect the child. Bluebond-Langer (1978) named this 'mutual pretence'. This engagement is a game, with each trying to protect the other, and can lead to the child feeling isolated and frightened. Kübler-Ross (1981) wrote that children who are facing death show little fear about it, but are more concerned about what will happen to their parents after they die. Spinetta (1982) challenges the 'protective' approach when considering talking to a child about impending death, as it is considered important that children are given the opportunity to talk about their worries and concerns while being offered appropriate support (Hindmarch 2000). An enhanced understanding can provide the child with a sense of control, which can in turn reduce fear as well as associated deleterious effects (Levetown and Committee of Bioethics 2008).

Knowing when to talk to children about death is difficult, and a number of factors have been suggested that warrant consideration before broaching the subject (AAP 2000). These include the child's disease experience and developmental level, the child's experience of death, the family's cultural and religious beliefs, and the child's patterns of coping as well as the expected circumstances regarding the death. Talking to children is often delayed while the parents themselves are learning about the diagnosis (Goldman 2000). However, as Hindmarch (2000) highlights, children will pick up instinctively that adults do not want to talk or show their feelings, and this delay can allow the child to misinterpret his or her own anxieties and delay coping (Black 1998).

Wolfe (2004) suggests the time to talk arrives when it is clear that the child knows something is wrong, and when the parents recognize the reality of the death occurring. Individuality is the key, and the unique needs and apparent direction desired by the child should be central. While children should have the opportunity to ask about death, if they refuse this they should not be forced into discussing it (Levetown and the Committee of Bioethics 2008). Siblings too have a need to talk about the impending death of their brother or sister. This gives them an opportunity to express their worries, have help to understand the situation and ease their adjustment in the bereavement period if they receive preparation (Lauer *et al.* 1985).

CLINICAL FOCUS

Mark is 12 years old and has had thirteen months of extensive treatment for a brain tumour. When the initial diagnosis was made, the interdisciplinary team talked with Mark's parents regarding how they felt about involving him in discussions about his illness. The parents always received the information first and then they explained it to Mark.

Mark's parents have just heard that all curative options have been exhausted and are frightened about discussing death with him. His friend, who also had a brain tumour, died three months earlier. The interdisciplinary team offer them explanations about awareness, while giving them support. The parents decide to take the lead from Mark and only mention it if he asks them. The team respect this and offers reassurance. They also make it clear that while they would not broach the subject with Mark, they would not lie to him if he asked them directly.

Preparations are under way to transfer Mark back home, where care is to be provided. The named nurse on the ward thinks Mark probably knows that he is dying and he has become quite withdrawn. The day before he goes home, when his Mum and the nurse are with him, he asks his Mum directly if he is going to die. His Mum is quite shaken and asks him why he thinks that; he says it is because everyone is very sad, and because he isn't having any more chemo. Mum explains that he is dying, and that no more treatment is available and everybody dies – some people when they are young, and some people when they are old, and then she describes heaven. Mum asks him what he is worrying about. Mark asks about pain and his concern about pain. They both cry and Mark says 'I didn't want to ask you because I knew it would make you cry again.'

APPLICATION IN PRACTICE

Applying the 6 Es strategy (Beale *et al.* 2006) to the care of Mark.

- **Establish**. The interdisciplinary team had established an agreement with the parents at the initial diagnosis and at the relapse stage about communicating with their son about death if he asked.

- **Engage**. The change in Mark's behaviour suggested that he was struggling with emotions. This and his direct question provided an opportunity for engaging in discussion.

- **Explore**. Mark's mother used questioning to explore what he already knew, and what he wanted to know about his condition. This permitted correction of any misconceptions and misunderstandings.

- **Explain**. Mark's mother gave an explanation to Mark based on his age and according to his desire for it. Reassurance regarding specific concerns, for example, about suffering pain, was given.

- **Empathise**. Crying with each other aided in showing empathy.

- **Encourage**. Encouragement was given to Mark by his mother reassuring him that he could talk and receive support as he required it.

This scenario demonstrates how the Beale *et al.* (2005) framework can guide discussion with children about death in practice. Importantly, Mark set the pace: his understanding was explored, his Mum listened to what he was saying, used simple language and clarified understanding. A dialogue with the child was encouraged and clearly illustrates what Hindmarch (2000) stresses as the importance of talking *with* the child as opposed to talking *to* the child. Honesty is important, as it is considered likely that if a child asks about his or her condition, there is already a suspicion that something is wrong and he/she is checking to see who they can trust (Levetown and the Committee of Bioethics 2008).

=== **WEB LINKS** ===

Resources can help parents to know how to talk to their children about death. Available at: www.cw.bc.ca/library/pdf/pamphlets/Talking%20About%20Death%20BCCH%201023.pdf Consider how a resource such as this could be developed and used in your practice.

In addition to imparting information to children (as outlined earlier in this chapter), play can help to break down barriers (Ellis 2000) by serving as a medium for the child and siblings expressing their fears, emotions and anxieties (Downs and Simons 2006). Play can act as a conduit to permit a connection between the child and professional, whilst promoting security and trust. It has been recognized that children are more likely to paint, talk or write about their emotions relating to illness, injury or even death, within a guided framework of play (Haiait et al. 2003). Play specialists and schoolteachers are pivotal members of the interdisciplinary team caring for the child with palliative care needs and, as such, can provide an environment where emotions can be expressed in a creative and therapeutic way.

The use of drawings has been commended as a useful method of communicating with dying children, siblings and bereaved children (Wellings 2001, Brown 2007). The aim of these approaches is to permit expressions of emotion and to foster positive attitudes (Rollins 2005). The psychologist, as part of the interdisciplinary team, can skilfully harness the power of drawing in prompting discussion with children and as a medium for expressing emotions.

Bluebond-Langer (1992) identified that parents are likely to be more open and honest with their child if adequate support is provided. Parents, therefore, should be guided and supported by the interdisciplinary team and helped to communicate with their children (including siblings) in a more open and honest way about illness, treatment and death (AAP 2000, Harrington Jacobs 2005). Hilden et al. (2000) stress how time and effort should be given to teaching and supporting families regarding talking to their children. Families also need reassurance about the benefits of an open approach with their children (Levetown and the Committee on Bioethics 2008).

KEY POINT

Parent's need guidance and support from the interdisciplinary team about talking to their children about death.

An important study by Kreicbergs et al. (2004) can guide practice within this difficult area. The quantitative study was carried out in Sweden and used questionnaires to establish whether parents had spoken to their child about his or her impending death; 429 parents out of 449 participants stated whether or not they had spoken to their child about death. None of the 147 parents who had talked about death regretted it, whereas 69 of 258 parents who did not talk about it regretted not having done so.

━━━━━━━━━━ **FURTHER READING** ━━━━━━━━━━

Read Kreicbergs *et al.* (2004) Talking about death with children who have severe malignant disease. *New England Journal of Medicine* **351**: 1175–86, and consider how the findings may help you in your work with parents who struggle with the decision of whether to discuss death with their child.

Despite being given support, guidance and information around the issue of truth-telling and talking to children about death, some families may still decide to withhold the truth from their child. The interdisciplinary team may feel torn, as conflict can ensue regarding what is best for the child versus the wishes of the parents.

The team caring for the child must respect the family's wishes and work in partnership with the family in a culture where openness and good communication is welcomed (Goldman 2007). Collaboration among the interdisciplinary team should create an atmosphere that fosters truthfulness (Dunlop 2008) and should ensure that the family are fully informed as to the knowledge that exists around the child's awareness of death.

Negotiating tensions and conflict

Tensions and conflicts can cause arguments between family members as well as between the family and the interdisciplinary team, given that emotions are heightened and families are stressed and anxious. Negotiation is important in solving problems and conflict, and must involve parents/child (if appropriate) and the interdisciplinary team striving towards a solution or joint decision about a problem (Matthews 2006).

━━━━━━━━━━ **ACTIVITY** ━━━━━━━━━━

Reflect on a situation in your practice where there was conflict between a parent and the interdisciplinary team member/members.

Consider how this was managed and think about alternative ways in which it might have been managed.

Conflict may be around truth-telling (as outlined above) or other aspects of care and care delivery, including decisions around DNR orders, commencing a syringe driver, withdrawing feeding, or changing place of care. While conflict can occur at any stage along the palliative care journey, it is more often discussed in the literature at critical junctures, particularly at the end-of-life.

Denial can cause tension, and it has been shown that professionals recognize the terminal phase of a child's illness a significant length of time before the parents do

(Wolfe *et al.* 2000). The notion of denial is further endorsed through the findings of an American study that examined attitudes and practices among paediatric oncologists regarding end-of-life care of children with regard to external forces which they saw as barriers to high quality care; 47.5 per cent cited an 'unrealistic expectation for cure' on the part of families; and 35.7 per cent identified family denial of the illness being terminal (Hilden *et al.* 2001). If families and professionals are not working together towards the same goals, then conflict may ensue.

While cases of extended unresolved conflict are not common, persistent disagreement can lead to the provision of inappropriate care to the child, to suffering and to a situation where distrust between the family and the interdisciplinary team is created (Masri *et al.* 2000). Despite having clear goals, managing emotions and understanding other perspectives, conflicts still arise (Feudtner 2007). Conflict should be openly addressed, and Feudtner (2007) identifies how often teams communicate while ignoring the root of the conflict. Lask (2003) stipulates that by accepting that conflict is a possibility within the therapeutic relationship, early recognition and resolution can be fostered. Toce (2001) suggests a medical consultation or an interdisciplinary team case conference as possible solutions to deal with conflict. Managing conflict is, therefore, an important skill, and most conflicts can be averted with high levels of communication between the interdisciplinary team and the family, anticipatory guidance and advanced care planning (Toce 2001).

Conclusion

The complexities involved in communicating with children and families have been outlined and discussed in this chapter. Clear, concise communication is surely the cornerstone of quality palliative care for children, and is the responsibility of every member of the interdisciplinary team. The individual and changing needs of the child and family require careful consideration and attention from those caring for the child and family. Professionals working within the speciality have expressed anxieties around communicating with families and parents of children who required palliative care further endorse the importance of communication, and the correlation between quality care and good levels of communication (Mack *et al.* 2005). The dichotomous relationship between communication and striving to offer the highest level of care possible to both children and their families, not only at the end-of-life but throughout the duration of the child's illness and life, is abundantly clear. With a sound knowledge base, support and clinical supervision, the different members of the interdisciplinary team can ensure expertise in communicating with children and families in an environment where openness and trust is created, and where children and families feel supported to express their fears and anxieties.

Key resources

ACT and RCPCH (Association for Children with Life-Threatening or Terminal Conditions and their Families) and The Royal College of Paediatrics and Child Health (2003) *A Guide to the Development of Children's Paediatric Services*, 2nd edn. Bristol: ACT.

Kaye, P. (1996) *Breaking Bad News (Pocket Book): A Ten Step Approach.* Northampton: EPL Publications.

Kreicbergs, U., Valdimarsdottir, U., Onelov, E., Henter, J., Steineck, G. (2004) Talking about death with children who have severe malignant disease. *New England Journal of Medicine* **351**: 1175–86.

CHAPTER SUMMARY

- High levels of communication are essential at the different stages along the palliative care journey.

- Communication in children's palliative care should be a partnership approach between the child (where appropriate), the family and the interdisciplinary team.

- A variety of communication skills should be adopted by the different members of the interdisciplinary team.

- A diverse range of communication tools are available when communicating with children: for example, play, art, story telling and so on.

- Good levels of communication and concise relevant information ensure that families are empowered to make decisions about care.

- Breaking bad news, decision-making, talking to children about death and meeting the information needs of children and families can be particularly challenging.

- Effective communication and quality care are inextricably linked.

Acknowledgement

The authors acknowledge the input of David Thomas, Lead Children's Oncology Macmillan Nurse Specialist, Leeds Teaching Hospitals NHS Trust, in the initial planning stage of this chapter.

References

ACT and RCPCH (Association for Children with Life-Threatening or Terminal Conditions and their Families and The Royal College of Paediatrics and Child Health) (2003) *A Guide to the Development of Children's Paediatric Services*, 2nd edn. Bristol: ACT.

ACT (Association for Children with Life-Threatening or Terminal Conditions and their Families) (2004a) *The ACT Charter for Children with Life-Threatening and Terminal Conditions and their Families.* Bristol: ACT. Available at www.act.org

ACT (Association for Children with Life-Threatening or Terminal Conditions and their Families) (2004b) *A Framework for the Development of Integrated Multi-Agency Care Pathways for Children with Life-Threatening and Life-Limiting Conditions.* Bristol: ACT. Available at: www.act.org.

American Academy of Pediatrics (AAP) (2000) Palliative care for children. *Pediatrics* **106**(2): 351–7.

Anghelescu, D., Oakes, L., and Hinds, P. (2006) Palliative care and pediatrics. *Anesthesiology Clinics of North America* **24**: 145–61.

Baile, W., Buckman, R., Lenzi, R., Glober, G., Beale, E. A., and Kudelka, A. P. (2000) SPIKES – A six-step protocol for delivering bad news: application to the patient with cancer. *The Oncologist* **5**: 302–11.

Beale, E. A., Baile, W. F. and Aaron, J. (2005) Silence is not golden: communicating with children dying from cancer. *Journal of Clinical Oncology*, **23**(15) (May 20): 3629–31.

Black, D. (1998) Coping with loss. The dying child. *BMJ* **316**: 1376–8

Blackburn, C. and Read, J. (2005) Using the internet? The experiences of parents with disabled children. *Child Care Health and Development* **31**(5): 507-15.

Bluebond-Langer, M. (1978) *Mutual Pretence: Causes and Consequences. The Private Worlds of Dying Children*, Princeton, NJ: Princeton University Press.

Bluebond-Langer, M. (1992) Chronically and terminally ill children: research directions for the 90's. *Loss, Grief and Care* **6**(1): 61–72.

Bradley, J. C. and Edinberg, M. A. (1982) *Communication in the Nursing Context*. Norwalk, CT: Appleton-Century-Crofts.

Brooks, W. and Heath, R. (1985) *Speech Communication*. 7th edn., Oxford: Madison.

Brown, E. (ed) (2007) *Supporting the Child and the Family in Paediatric Palliative Care*. London: Jessica Kingsley.

Buckman, R. (1992) *Breaking Bad News: A Guide for Healthcare Professionals*. Baltimore, MD: Johns Hopkins University Press.

Clarke, J. and Fletcher, P. (2003) Communication issues faced by parents who have a child diagnosed with cancer. *Journal of Pediatric Oncology Nursing* **20**(4):173–91.

Contro, N., Larson, J., Schofield, S., Sourkes, B. and Cohen, H. (2002) Family perspectives on the quality of pediatric palliative care. *Archives of Pediatric Adolescent Medicine* **156**: 14–19.

Contro, N., Larson, J., Schofield, S., Sourkes, B. and Cohen, H. (2004) Hospital staff and family perspectives regarding quality of pediatric palliative care. *Pediatrics* **114**(5): 1248–52.

Cooley, C. (2000) Communication skills in palliative care. *Professional Nurse* **15**(9): 603-5.

Cooley, C. (2005) Communication skills in palliative care. In Faull, C., Carter, Y. and Daniels, L. (eds) *Handbook of Palliative Care* (2nd edn). Oxford: Blackwell.

Costello, J. and Trinder-Brook, A. (2000) Children's nurses' experiences of caring for dying children in hospital. *Paediatric Nursing* **12**(6): 28–32.

Coulter, A., Entwistle, V. and Gilbert, D. (1999) Sharing decisions with patients: is the information good enough? *British Medical Journal* **318**: 318–22.

Davies, B. and Connaughty, S. (2002) Pediatric end-of-life care: lessons learned from parents. *Journal of the American Medical Association* **32**(1): 5–6.

DHSSPS (Department of Health, Social Services and Public Safety) (2003) *Breaking Bad News Regional Guidelines*. Belfast: HMSO.

Dighe, M., Jadhav, S., Muckaden, M. A. and Sovani, A. (2008) Parental concerns in children requiring palliative care. *Indian Journal of Palliative Care* **14**(1): 16–22.

Done, A. (2001) The therapeutic use of story telling. *Paediatric Nursing* **13**(3): 17–20.

Downs, G. and Simons, J. (2006) Communication. In: Goldman, A., Hain, R. and Liben, S. (eds) *Oxford Textbook of Palliative Care for Children*. Oxford: Oxford University Press, pp. 28–41.

Dunlop, S. (2008) The dying child: should we tell the truth? *Paediatric Nursing* **20**: 828–31.

Ellis, J. (2000) Games without frontiers. *Nursing Times* **96**(26): 32–3.

Feudtner, C. (2007) Collaborative communication in pediatric palliative care: a foundation for problem-solving and decision-making. *Pediatric Clinics of North America* **54**: 583–607.

Foster, T. L. (2007) Pediatric palliative care revisited: a vision to add life. *Journal of Hospice and Palliative Nursing* **9**(4): 212–19.

GMC (General Medical Council) (2006) *Good Medical Practice. Guidelines for Doctors and 0–18 years: Guidance to for All Doctors*, Part 14. Available at: www.gmc-uk.org/guidance/archive/GMC_0–18.pdf

Goldman, A. (2000) Palliative care for children. In Faull, C., Carter, Y. and Woolf, R. (eds) *Handbook of Palliative Care*. Oxford: Blackwell Science, ch. 16, pp. 256–71.

Goldman, A. (2007) An overview of paediatric palliative care. *Medical Principles and practices* **16** (Supp. 1): 46–7.

Haitait, H., Bar-Mor, G., Schobat, M. (2003) The world of the child: a world of play even in hospital. *Journal of Pediatric Nursing* **18**(3): 209–14.

Harrington Jacobs, H. (2005) Ethics in pediatric end-of-life care: a nursing perspective. *Journal of Pediatric Nursing* **20**(5): 360–9.

Hewitt-Taylor, J. (2005) Caring for children with complex and continuing health needs. *Nursing Standard* **19**(42): 41–7.

Hewitt-Taylor, J. (2008) Parents' views of their children who have complex health needs. *Paediatric Nursing* **20**(8): 20–3.

Hilden, J., Watterson, J. and Chrastek. J. (2000) Tell the children. *Journal of Clinical Oncology* **18**(17): 3193–5.

Himelstein, B. P. (2006) Palliative care for infants, children, adolescents and their families. *Journal of Palliative Medicine* **9**(1): 163–78.

Hindmarch, C. (2000) On the death of a child. Oxford: Radcliffe Medical Press.

Hinds, P., Drew, D., Oakes, L., Fouladi, M., Spunt, S., Church, C. and Furman, W. (2005) End-of-life care preferences of pediatric patients with cancer. *Journal of Clinical Oncology* **36**(9): 9146–54.

Hummelinck, A. and Pollock, K. (2006) Parents' information needs about treatment of their chronically ill child: a qualitative study. *Patient Education and Counseling* **62**: 228–34.

Hynson, J., Gillis, J., Collins, J., Irving, H. and Trethewie, J. (2003) The dying child: how is care different? *Medical Journal of Australia* **179**: S20–S22.

ICPCN (International Children's Palliative Care Network) (2008) *The ICPCN Charter of Rights for Life Limited and Life Threatened Children.* Available at: www.icpcn.org.uk/page.asp?section=000100010014&sectionTitle=Charter

IMPaCCT (2007) IMPaCCT: standards for paediatric palliative care in Europe. *European Journal of Palliative Care* **14**(3): 2–7.

James, L. and Johnson, B. (1997) The needs of parents of pediatric oncology patients during the palliative care phase. *Journal of Pediatric Oncology Nursing* **14**(2): 83–95.

Judd, D. (1998) Communicating with dying children. In Dickenson, D. and Johnson, M. (eds) *Death, Dying and Bereavement.* London/Newbury Park, CA: Sage/Open University.

Kane, J. R., Brown Hellsten, M, Coldsmith, A. (2004) Human suffering: the need for relationship-based research in pediatric end-of-life care. *Journal of Pediatric Oncology Nursing* **21**(3): 180–5.

Kaye, P. (1996) *Breaking Bad News (Pocket Book): A Ten Step Approach.* Northampton: EPL Publications.

Kenyon, B. (2001) Current research in children's conceptions of death: a critical review. *The Journal of Death and Dying* **43**(1): 69–91.

Kolarik, R. C., Walker, G., Arnold, R. M. (2006) Pediatric resident education in palliative care: a needs assessment. *Pediatrics* **117**: 1949–54.

Kreicbergs, U., Valdimarsdottir, U. , Onelov, E., Henter, J., Steineck, G. (2004) Talking about death with children who have severe malignant disease. *New England Journal of Medicine* **351**: 1175–86.

Kübler-Ross, E. (1970) *On Death and Dying.* New York: Macmillan.

Kübler-Ross, E. (1981) *Living with Death and Dying.* New York: Macmillan.

Kuttner, L. (2007) Talking with families when their children are dying. *Medical Principles and Practice* **16** (Suppl. 1): 16–20.

Lansdown, R. (1994) Communication with children. In Goldman, A. (ed) *Care of the Dying Child.* Oxford: Oxford University Press.

Langton, H. (ed.) (2000) *The Child with Cancer – Family-centred Care in Practice.* Edinburgh: Bailliere Tindall.

Larcher, V. (2006) Ethics. In Goldman, A., Hain, R. and Liben, S. (eds) *Oxford Textbook of Palliative Care for Children*. Oxford: Oxford University Press, pp. 42–59.

Lask, B. (2003) Patient–clinician conflict: causes and compromises. *Journal of Cystic Fibrosis* **2**: 42–5.

Lauer, M. E., Mulhern, R. K., Bohne, E. B., and Camitta, B. M. (1985) Children's perceptions of their sibling's death at home or in hospital: the precursors to differential adjustment. *Cancer Nursing* **8**: 21–7.

Levetown, M. and the Committee on Bioethics (2008) Communicating with children and families: from everyday interactions to skill in conveying distressing symptoms. *Pediatrics* **121**: 1441–60.

Mack, J. W., Hilden, J. M., Watterson, J., Moore, C., Turner, B., Grier, H., Weeks, J. and Wolfe, J. (2005) Parent and physician perspectives on quality of care at the end of life in children with cancer. *Journal of Clinical Oncology* **23**: 9162–71.

McNeilly, P., Price, J. and McCloskey, S. (2006) Reflection in children's palliative care: a model. *European Journal of Palliative Care* **13**(1): 31–4.

Masri, C. , Farrell, C. A., Lacroix, J. (2000) Decision making and end-of-life care in critically ill care. *Journal of Palliative Care Supplement*: S45–S52.

Matthews, J. (2006) Communicating with children and their families. In Glasper, A. and Richardson, J. (eds) *A Textbook of Children's and Young People's Nursing*. London: Elsevier, ch. 10.

Meyer, E. C., Ritholz, M. D., Burns, J. P. and Truog, R. D. (2006) Improving the quality of end-of-life care in the pediatric intensive care unit: parents' priorities and recommendations. *Pediatrics* **117**(3): 649–57.

Molen, van der, B. (2007) Providing patient information – Part 1: Assessing information needs of patients. *European Journal of Cancer Care* **16**: 312.

Nagy, M. (1948) The child's theories concerning death. *The Journal of Genetic Psychology* **73**: 3–27.

Patterson Kelly, K. and Porock, D. (2005) A survey of pediatric oncology nurses' perceptions of patients' educational needs. *Journal of Pediatric Oncology Nursing* **22**(1): 58–66.

Peel, N. (2003) The role of the critical care nurse in the delivery of bad news. *British Journal of Nursing* **12**(16): 966–71.

Price, J. (2003) Information needs of the child with cancer and their family. *Cancer Nursing Practice* **2**(7): 35–8.

Price, J. and McFarlane, M. (2006) Care of the child requiring palliative care. In Glasper, E. A. and Richardson, J. (eds) *Children and Young People's Nursing*. Oxford: Elsevier.

Price, J. and Spence, N. (2004) Play in the community – quality care for the child with cancer. *Cancer Nursing Practice* **38**: 31–4.

Price, J., McNeilly, P. and Surgenor, M. (2006) Breaking bad news to parents – the children's nurse's role. *International Journal of Palliative Nursing* **12**(3): 115–20.

RCPCH (Royal College of Paediatrics and Child Health) (2004) *Withholding or Withdrawing Life Sustaining Treatment in Children: A Framework for Practice*, 2nd edn. London: RCPCH.

Rollins, J. (2005) Tell me about it: drawing as a communication tool for children with cancer. *Journal of Pediatric Oncology* **22**(4): 203–21.

Rushton, C. H. (2005) A framework for integrated pediatric palliative care: being with dying. *Journal of Pediatric Nursing* **20**(5): 311–23.

Spinetta, J. J. (1982) Behavioural and psychological research in childhood cancer: an overview. *Cancer* **50**: 1939–43.

Stark, C. (2003) *The New Medical Conversation: Media, Patients, Doctors, and the Ethics of Scientific Communication*. Book Review. *British Medical Journal* **327**: 755.

Starke, M. and Mollers, A. (2002) Parents' needs for knowledge concerning the medical diagnosis of their children. *Journal of Child Health Care* **6**: 245–57.

Steele, R. (2002) Experiences of families in which a child has a prolonged terminal illness: modifying factors. *International Journal of Palliative Nursing* **8**(9): 418–34.

Stevens, M. (1996) Psychological adaptation of the dying child. In Doyle, D., Hanks, G. and Macdonald, N. (eds) *Oxford Textbook of Palliative Medicine*. Oxford: Oxford University Press, pp. 699–70

Thornes, R. (2001) Palliative care for young people aged 13–24. Joint Working Party on Palliative Care for Adolescents and Young People. Available at: www.library.nhs.uk/childhealth/View Resource.aspx?resID=259729

Thurgate, C. (2006) Living with disability. Part 3: Communication and care. *Paediatric Nursing*. **18**(5): 38–44.

Toce, S. (2001) Ethical decision making for the child with a life-limiting condition. *Supportive Voice* **7**: 4.

Twycross, R. (2003) *Introducing Palliative Care*. Oxford: Radcliffe Medical Press.

Wainstein, B, K., Sterling-Levis, Baker, S. A., Taitz, J. and Brydon, M. (2006) Use of Internet by parents of paediatric patients. *Journal of Paediatrics and Child Health* **42**(9): 528–32.

Wellings, T. (2001) Drawings by dying and beareaved families. *Paediatric Nursing* **13**(4): 30–6.

WMPMT (West Midlands Paediatric Macmillan Team) (2005) *Palliative Care for Children with Malignant Disease*. London: Quay Books.

Wolfe, J., Klar, N., Grier, H. E., Duncan, J., Salem-Schatz, S., Emanuel, E. J. and, Weeks, J.C. (2000) Understanding of prognosis among parents of children who died of cancer: impact on treatment goals and integration of palliative care. *Journal of the American Medical Association* **284**(19): 2469–75.

Wolfe, L. (2004) Should parents speak with a dying child about impending death? *The New England Journal of Medicine* **351**: 1251–3.

Young, B., ,Dixon-Woods, M., Windridge, K. and Heney, D. (2003) Managing communication with young people who have a potentially life threatening chronic illness: qualitative study of patients and parents. *British Medical Journal* **326**(Feb): 305.

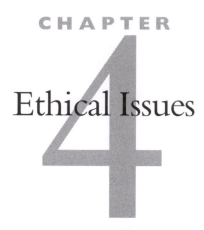

CHAPTER 4

Ethical Issues

Helen Bennett

Introduction

Moral and ethical issues are embedded in all aspects of health and social care practice. Advancing medical technology, developing evidenced-based practice and the nature of childhood conditions in palliative care means that the choices and options for parents and families have become wider and more diverse. The increasing complexity of care provision means that ethical dilemmas are not always straightforward, and the challenges for practitioners in decision-making are increasingly complex.

An awareness of the law, the legal aspects of care and underpinning ethical principles are therefore essential to achieve effective decision-making. Alongside our developing understanding of children's and families' experiences, it is clear that decision-making in palliative care requires an ethical approach encompassing all the dimensions of care that influence the illness journey.

The purpose of this chapter is to address the key ethical dilemmas and debates in children's palliative care practice, and offer an approach to ethical decision-making that meets the individual experiences of children and their families.

KEY POINT

With developing technology and multiple choices of treatment for children with life-threatening conditions, ethical issues in practice are becoming wider and more diverse.

Legal aspects

The relationship between the law and ethics or morals is complex, being both intertwined and separate (Hope *et al.* 2003). Within children's palliative care, the interface of legal aspects of care is equally challenging, in particular around consent to treatment for children. At such a difficult and emotive time, and when the risks can be great, this has a further impact on the decision-making process. Yet an awareness and understanding of the law is essential to our knowledge of ethics.

There is a wealth of literature written on children's law and the legal dimensions of child health care (Hendrick 2000, Dimond 2002). These texts address in full the application of the law, and the challenges and conflicts that arise in child health care. It is not the intention of this chapter to repeat this work. Nevertheless, there are aspects of the law that explicitly affect the issues that arise in children's palliative care and ethical decision-making, and these will be drawn on to provide evidence for debate.

There are a number of key acts and principles underpinning children's palliative care practice – these are listed and summarized in Figure 4.1.

Parental responsibility

Parental responsibility is a legal concept encompassing the rights, duties, powers, responsibilities and authority that most parents have towards their children. Such responsibility includes the right of parents to consent to medical treatment for their children, though this right is not absolute (BMA 2008). Parental responsibility is granted with the understanding that parents will act in the best interests of their children. With the growing capacity of a child's competence, however, parental responsibility decreases (see section Principles of autonomy, competence and consent, below).

A recent revision in the law regarding parental responsibility refers to equal responsibility of both parents if registered on the birth certificate after 1 December 2003 (England and Wales), 15 April 2002 (Northern Ireland) or 6 May 2006 (Scotland). This applies irrespective of whether the parents are married. Prior to these dates, a child's biological parents will only automatically acquire parental responsibility if they were married at the time of the child's conception or at some time thereafter. If unmarried, the father may acquire responsibility by applying via a parental responsibility agreement from the court.

Rights of the child

The basic rights of the child are reflected in the United Nations Convention on the Rights of the Child (UNCRC) (see Figure 4.1) and have laid the foundations for the promotion of children's rights in the UK. It is often held up as the most significant influencing factor in the development of the framework allowing children to participate in decisions affecting their lives (Fajerman *et al.* 2004). The fundamental principles of autonomy, freedom of expression and choice underpinning children's rights are also recognized in *Every Child Matters* (DH 2003) and the

The Family Law Reform Act (DH 1969) Emphasized parental responsibility of Children to the age of 18 but acknowledged the right to consent for children aged 16 or 17 independently of their parents. However, the refusal of treatment can be overruled.

The Children Act England and Wales (DH 1989) The Children Act emphasizes the safety and welfare of all children, and states that the views of the child should be heard.

The Children Act (1995) Scotland and Northern Ireland Children Order (1995) Alongside the UK this Act was a major piece of legislation and emphasized that the views of the child must be taken into account.

United Nations Convention on the Rights of the Child (United Nations 1989) This was ratified by UK government and requires the government to honour the convention and its recommendations to respect the rights of all children. In particular, Article 12 states that children and young people should have the opportunity to express their views on matters that concern them, and to have those views taken into account when decisions are made.

The Human Rights Act (DH 2000) Overall, the Human Rights Act aims to protect individual freedom with a number of articles relevant to health care that are transferable to children.

Every Child Matters (DH 2003) This Department of Health Green Paper and the recommendations for change to the children's service, was a response to the inadequacies highlighted in the Victoria Climbie report (Lord Laming). The paper sets out a range of measures to reform children's care across England and Wales. It gives particular attention to the health and well being of all children, and the provision of services for children to maximize and achieve their full potential.

The Children Act (DH 2004a) Building on the previous Children Act (1989), emphasizes the importance of a children's commissioner who has responsibility for the welfare of children in England and Wales in promoting the children's views and interests. In addition, it establishes a duty on local authorities to provide coherent and comprehensive children's services.

The National Service Framework for Children, Young People and Maternity Services (2004b) This NSF is a ten-year programme aimed at stimulating a long-term and sustained improvement in children's health. In particular, Standard 8 recognizes the development of co-ordinated high-quality services for disabled children and young people and those with complex health needs.

The Mental Capacity Act (DH 2005b) While this is primarily for adults, it does affect young people aged 16 and over. The act addresses issues in relation to capacity and decision-making.

The Convention on the Rights of Persons with Disabilities (United Nations 2007) The Convention on the Rights of Persons with Disabilities opened for signature in March 2007 has heralded a breakthrough for disabled adults and children alike. Article 7 (para. 3) of this convention focuses on the right of children with disabilities to express their views and be provided with appropriate assistance in order to do this. Hence this treaty specifically addresses the voices of disabled children and the mechanisms required to ensure that their voices are heard.

Better Care: Better Lives (DH 2008) This strategy sets the future direction for children's palliative care services. The document further highlights key recommendations to provide equitable access to high- quality family- centred sustainable care.

Figure 4.1 Key acts and principles underpinning children's palliative care practice

National Service Framework for Children, Young People and Maternity Services (DH 2004b). However, the degree to which children have a voice and are encouraged to participate is still hampered by interpretations of childhood (Lowden 2002) and a lack of acknowledgement of a child's capacity and ability to contribute to decision-making.

The National Children's Bureau (2008) and Save the Children (2008) actively work in promoting children's rights and participation, and emphasize the consideration of the rights of the child in all aspects of health care.

Fajerman *et al* (2004), while recognizing children's rights derived from the UNCRC (1989), recommend guiding principles for children's participation and consultation, including:

- Children's right to be listened to and to freely express their views.

- Equal right to participation.

- Measures in place to encourage and facilitate their participation in accordance with their age and maturity.

- Participation that promotes the best interests of the child and enhances personal development.

The United Nations Convention on the Rights of Persons with Disability also addresses the rights and protection of children with a disability (Article 7) promoting equal rights with other children (United Nations, 2008).

ACTIVITY

Consider the guidance and recommendations from any of these Acts and DH papers, and describe how they are or can be integrated in to your practice area, taking in to account parental responsibility and the rights of the child.

Context of ethics

The depth of debate in health care ethics has grown considerably since the 1980s, and the moral issues raised in palliative care are clearly evident (Randall and Downie 1999, Casarett 2005). Much has been discussed surrounding ethical issues at the end of life; for example, euthanasia and assisted suicide, though mainly from an adult perspective. The focus of debate for children has centred on consent (Alderson 1992), competence to consent (Friedman Ross 2001, Wheeler 2006), the child's contribution to and participation in decision-making (BMA 2001), and the withdrawal and withholding of life-prolonging treatment (RCPCH 2004).

Discussion given to the process for decision-making has drawn predominately on the traditional principle-based approach to ethics (Ashcroft 2007). It is widespread practice to address underpinning principles such as competence, consent and autonomy, and indeed these are discussed in depth (Alderson 1992, 1995; BMA 2001). However, while these principles have their place in medical decision–making, the ethical challenges of children's palliative care requires further attention to understand the context of the child's and family's experience.

Approaches to ethics

In order to address the ethical issues faced in children's palliative care and to promote active participation in the decision-making process, an understanding of the ethical approaches that define our thinking are essential to support good ethical practice. The wider aspects of care, including teamwork, partnership and attention to detail within the child and family relationship, are critical. The individual constructs of the child and childhood are also important dimensions to consider, a perspective that is often missing.

Traditional approaches to ethics have focused on the four principles of autonomy, beneficence, non-maleficence and justice (Beauchamp and Childress 2001) (see Figure 4.2). However, it is argued that this approach cannot support the diversity of health care ethics (Ashcroft 2007), and there is significant pressure to promote other ways of ethical thinking (Feudtner 2007).

When applying solely a principle-based approach, conflict can arise; for example, supporting the autonomy of the child versus the rights of the parents. This tension cannot easily be resolved by the application of rules and principles, and a more sensitive exploration of the situation is needed in order to understand the complex nature of decision-making in children's palliative care.

In contrast to the four principles (Beauchamp and Childress 2001) there are a number of approaches that consider a more value-based and relational approach to ethics (Woods 2001) emphasizing the importance of collaborative communication (Feudtner 2007). A feminist and situated ethical approach, which accentuates the context of children's palliative care practice, provides an additional perspective. Feminist ethics stresses the importance of individual values, with an

---

Autonomy: self-determination, the ability to decide and act on one's own thoughts freely and independently. A child has a right to be autonomous, and if not competent, to have their views and interests taken into consideration. They should be involved and be able to express freely their choices in health care.

Beneficence: the moral obligation to do good. This principle reflects the best interests of the child and that we should always balance the benefits and harms of treatment to promote the best outcome for the child.

Non-maleficence: to do no harm. The benefits of treatment should outweigh the risks. If the potential harm is considered to be too great, then treatment can be withheld or withdrawn.

Justice: to be fair and equitable. The distribution of resources and access to children's palliative care services is central to this principle

---

Figure 4.2   Key acts and principles underpinning children's palliative care practice

Source: Beauchamp and Childress (2001).

Guidelines for ethical thinking

- Who is involved and affected by the ethical dilemma?
- What is the context the situation and available knowledge?
- What are the social and personal elements?
- What are the needs of those involved?
- What is your role within the situation?
- What is the balance of personal and social power of those involved?
- How will those involved understand the actions and consequences?
- Are these in balance with our own judgements?
- How can we best communicate with all those involved?

Figure 4.3 Guidelines for ethical thinking

Source: Adapted from Edwards and Mauthner (2002).

emphasis on care and relationships. Situated ethics is about how ethics are constructed and practised , and takes into account the cultural and societal dimensions influencing the issues that arise.

Integrating such an approach considers the differences that children and families experience. It acknowledges the way that individuals talk about their lives, and how they make sense of them. These values are crucial in underpinning palliative care practice, and for supporting the child and family throughout the illness journey. For children, we must recognize the multiple perspectives and views of the child throughout childhood. From a care perspective it enables greater attention to be given to the child within the family context. It reinforces the importance of the child's experience, age and development, and the impact this has on their capacity to participate in decisions about their care. Therefore, emphasis on collaborative communication between health care professionals, the child and family is essential (Feudtner 2007), as it helps professionals to recognize the need to support the child in developing relationships and key personal values (Alderson 1995).

In order to promote and develop sensitive communication and to understand the relationships involved, there are aspects of ethical thinking that are helpful to consider (see Figure 4.3).

ACTIVITY

Reflect on an ethical dilemma in practice, and describe what elements you need to consider in order to further understand the situation.

Decision-making

It is well recognized in children's health care that a tripartite relationship between child, parent and health care professional is essential for effective decision-making.

In addition, it is increasingly acknowledged that children have much to contribute when it comes to issues of their own health (Baston 2008).

This relationship and recognition of the child's involvement in children's palliative care practice is pivotal to decision-making. However, while complex ethical problems are not common in child health care, the emotional impact and uncertainty for many living with a child with a life- limiting or threatening condition can make decision-making more difficult (McConnell *et al.* 2004). Effective and meaningful approaches to decision-making are therefore crucial in promoting and providing a way to include all those affected by a decision.

Fundamental aspects for decision-making, including collaborative communication, best interests, competence and consent, are addressed throughout the literature (BMA 2001, Lowden 2002, Alderson 2005, Feudtner 2007, Baston 2008) (see the section on Principles of autonomy, competence and consent below) and guidelines are presented by way of supporting the decision-making process. Hinds *et al.* (2001), following a study with adolescents, parents and health care providers, specifically recommend guidelines for decision-making at the end of life (see Clinical focus and guidelines for decision-making below).

In addition, Woods (2001) and Feudtner (2007) reinforce the importance of communication and dialogue to engage parents (and children) more fully in the choices and decisions of the dilemma that will lead to the best care possible and an acceptable moral outcome.

However, there will be occasions of conflict and disagreement, and it may never be simple to find an adequate solution (Woods 2001), particularly surrounding complex decisions in palliative and end-of-life care situations. Most commonly cited is the conflict between the child's rights and best interest, and parental responsibility and the role of advocacy. Parents have identified that end-of-life decisions are the most difficult they have to make (Hinds *et al.* 1997). In addition, health care professionals have stated that they feel inadequately prepared to assist parents with such difficult decisions (Hinds *et al.* 2001). This indicates a recognized need for professional development and training in end-of-life decision-making to enable professionals to better communicate with and support children and families with difficult choices to make. Furthermore, recent discussions suggest it is not about taking sides, but rather about promoting a culture where ethical dilemmas can be openly addressed. Consideration can be given to the whole situation, with acknowledgement of the values and views of all involved.

Throughout the decision-making process it is essential to maintain open and honest communication and to know that, if disagreement remains unresolved, the courts may be involved (BMA 2001).

KEY POINT

Attention to effective communication and the relationship between the child, parents and professionals is important to promote sensitive, meaningful decision-making.

CLINICAL FOCUS

Sam is a 12-year-old boy with spinal muscular atrophy type II. He is presenting with deteriorating respiratory function. He is very breathless, restless, has disturbed sleep, waking with headaches and feeling extremely tired. He is currently in the children's hospice for planned respite care.

Sam and his family have been known to the care team in the hospice for the past six years and have noticed a general deterioration in his condition. Sam's changing symptoms are assessed and a symptom management plan is now being implemented. Given this rapid deterioration, the care team feel that it is time to raise the issue of resuscitation with the family should Sam continue to decline.

The interdisciplinary team have planned to meet the family to discuss how best to manage this changing situation and to address the ongoing care needs and support for both Sam and his family.

APPLICATION IN PRACTICE

Key points to consider in decision-making; adapted from Gibson (1993) Hinds *et al.* (2001)

- Recognize the dilemma/situation and understand the wider contextual issues (focusing on a situated ethical approach).

- Actively seek opportunities to provide appropriate information (essential elements of informed consent).

- Provide opportunities to include and hear the views of all involved (autonomy and rights) – decision-making is a shared responsibility between the child, family and health care professionals (understanding the relationships involved within a feminist ethical approach will enhance understanding of the situation).

- Promote open and honest communication to aid decision-making and provide clear explanations.

- Health care professionals should understand the options available and any alternative treatments/care, consequences and long-term outcomes (to weigh up the risks and benefits and seek the best available individual outcome for the child and family).

- Document and inform other team members of the outcome of the conversation/decision (teamwork and partnership is essential to provide effective care).

- The health care team should be available to the child and family for further discussion and to deal with any related concerns (sensitive ongoing care will help continuous attention to treatment and care options).

- Provide the opportunity for evaluation, review and reflection (the value of learning from reflective practice to improve care for children and families)

ACTIVITY

In what ways can you facilitate the involvement of children in decision-making in practice?

The development of children's rights can also be addressed through understanding the principles of autonomy, competence and consent for children.

Principles of autonomy, competence and consent

Autonomy

The principle of autonomy demands that individuals including children have a right to freedom and choice (UNCRC 1989, NCB 2008, Fajerman *et al.* 2004) and to have their choices respected. The concept of autonomy is grounded in the belief that, to be autonomous, an individual should also have the capacity to decide and understand the consequences of the choices made. It is intrinsically linked to the concepts of competence and consent.

If autonomy is assessed on this basis, there are many who believe that children, if given relevant explanations, are capable of being autonomous, given time (Alderson 1992, Alderson and Montgomery 1996, BMA 2001). Yet the ability of children to participate and make autonomous decisions in relation to their health care has provided long-standing debate (Leikin 1993, Broome 1999). The focus of debate and conflict centres on a child's competence and his or her capacity to decide.

Competence

Competence implies that a person is mentally capable of understanding the nature and purpose of the decision being made, together with the possible outcomes and consequences. The limitation of assessing and measuring competence in children (Friedman Ross 2001) raises significant debate.

The standard measure recognized in law is that of age. However, it is argued that measuring competence by age alone is unreliable (Wheeler 2006). In addition, defining adulthood by age is not always clear. Assessment of competence should therefore also take into account a child's development, cognitive ability and experience (Alderson 1992). For 16-year-olds this is reinforced by the Mental Capacity Act (DH, 2005b), which addresses capacity and decision-making for young people aged 16–17 years.

In addition, Foster (2001) highlights the importance of and the risk involved in the decision to be made when assessing competence. This is central to decision-making in palliative care. Children may be considered competent and therefore autonomous to make low- risk decisions, but with complex decisions are less likely to be fully autonomous, because of lack of experience and capacity to understand the consequences. For example, a child may not be able to make a competent decision regarding the need for intravenous antibiotics for a chest infection, but would be able to choose in which arm they want the cannula.

It is perhaps assumed that a greater level of competence is required to validate a child's consent or not to treatment within palliative care. Conversely, it is argued that rather than requiring a greater level of competence, there is a need to provide more detailed information within the context of treatment (Alderson 2005). Any new situation requires a more in-depth explanation and the issues of complexity and uncertainty in the decision may be no greater for children than for adults. It is therefore not just about measuring competence, but rather a way of relating to children to understand their views and experiences (Alderson 1992).

━━━━━━━━━━━━━━━ **ACTIVITY** ━━━━━━━━━━━━━━━

List the types of autonomous decisions you would expect a 14-year-old young man with Duchenne muscular dystrophy would make, and those decisions for which you would expect to seek support from his parents. Explain your rationale using the information from this chapter.

Consent

In general terms, consent is valid when given voluntarily (freely), when the individual is fully informed and understands the consequences. The legal age of consent in England and Wales is 18 (Children Act 1989). The Family Law Reform Act (1969) respects consent to treatment at age 16, but not refusal, and if a child refuses treatment his/her decision can be overturned. The Mental Capacity Act (DH, 2005b), while reinforcing capacity for decision-making for 16-year-olds, states that only those over 18 can make an advance decision to refuse medical treatment.

Despite legal guidelines, the criterion of age to measure ability to consent has been criticized openly (Eiser 1990). Eiser claims that developmental level may be more appropriate, as it is the child's capacity to consent that is important in their ability to consent, rather than his or her age. In addition, Eiser (1990) and Alderson (1992) argue that a child's ability to consent should be understood in relation to the wider contextual factors, social and cultural influences. This distinction in promoting capacity to consent was influenced significantly by the Gillick case (1983), which acknowledged that, irrespective of age, a child who has the capacity to fully understand the implications of his or her decision could give valid consent – a criterion known as the 'Gillick test' (1985).

Informed consent requires comprehensive information to be given to the child, applicable to their age and understanding, and is a requirement in health care equal to that of providing information to adults (RCN 2006). However, the level of information required that is appropriate for a child to understand is uncertain (Burns 2003) and means that children are often excluded from participating in decisions. Alderson (2005) suggests that children have been excluded from decision-making on the grounds that they are not fully able to grasp all the information necessary to participate or consent. This is evident in children's palliative care, whereby a child may be able to consent to treatment without fully understanding the long-term consequences of their condition. However, it is an assumed interpretation of a child's understanding, and to date there is limited evidence and knowledge to support such a view. The responsibility lies with the health care professional to explore the child's understanding and to communicate appropriately in order to enable him/her to consent.

If children are unable to consent, it is important that assent is sought (Hendrick 2000). Assent should still be informed, willing and with co-operation from the child. It enables the child to indicate his/her opinions and wishes, and a right to receive information in a way that he or she can understand. This is required for all aspects of care and treatment.

Both assent and consent need to be perceived as an ongoing process of information-giving and expression of views (Morrow and Richards 1996). The debate surrounding consent and competence for children is ongoing and the challenges for practitioners remain.

Parental consent

One way in which consent is approached is through parental consent (supported within the Family Law Reform Act 1969) on the basis that parents have responsibility for their child and will act in its best interests. The requirement for parental consent is still largely influenced by the law rather than left to the consideration of the practitioner. Furthermore, obtaining parental consent is a necessary caution following the Alder Hey organs scandal and Bristol incident during the 1980s and 1990s, where parental consent was not sought. The increasing number of safeguards in health care settings to protect children and their families reflects a raised awareness of child protection issues in which parental consent offers some security within health care delivery. Yet, it is argued that a child who is able to understand the nature and consequences of the decisions being taken and has the capacity to decide should be able to do so without parental consent. As a way to resolve this tension, Dimond describes the process of parallel consent, to gain the views of both parent and child (Dimond 2002).

Consent in palliative care raises further dilemmas associated with capacity to consent because of the nature of the illness, the complexity of treatment and uncertainty around the end of life. Attention to continuous consent is important, and the opportunity to revisit and review consent at any time (Addington-Hall 2002).

FURTHER READING

Read Baston J. (2008) Healthcare decisions: a review of children's involvement. *Paediatric Nursing* **20**(3): 24–6. Consider recent changes to the ways in which we are encouraged to involve children in decision-making.

Truth-telling

Disclosure of information (which includes the 'breaking of bad news') and truth-telling (veracity) is often discussed in relation to the doctor patient relationship (Tuckett 2004, Higgs 2007). In children's palliative care, we refer to truthfulness within the tripartite relationship between the child, the family and the interdisciplinary team.

On the whole, truthfulness is considered best practice and it is generally assumed that patients want to know the truth. This is no different for children, not least when it is recognized that children with a life- threatening illness are aware of their condition and impending death.

The issue of truth-telling with children remains controversial, and the dilemmas are not easily resolved, with consistently strong arguments both for and against truth-telling.

For practitioners working within these sometimes difficult and emotive circumstances, it is not always easy to find an acceptable outcome that meets the values of all involved. However, respecting the values and beliefs of the child and family within the context of the family, encouraging effective communication and partnership working will establish a culture of openness where such dilemmas can be addressed.

Long-term ventilation

There is a growing population of children who are supported with long-term ventilation (LTV) (Jardine *et al.* 1999, Pfund 2007). Long-term ventilation is offered to any child who is medically stable but continues to require medical aid for breathing after an acknowledged failure to wean or is slow to wean after commencing ventilation (DH 2005a).

However, the uncertainty of whether a child with palliative care needs should receive long-term ventilation raises a number of ethical questions. The associated difficulty in relation to children's palliative care surrounds the trajectory of a number of conditions. The very nature of a degenerative illness means the child is unlikely to remain medically stable. There is also a lack of evidence and limited knowledge of the long-term consequences of LTV in children with life-threatening conditions. Heaton *et al.* (2003) highlight the demands of frequent hospital visits, availability of respite, and of educational and social isolation. Further issues arise around the impact of resources, funding and provision of collaborative partnerships to support children and families in the community.

In contrast, all children have the right to high-quality, high standards of care (DH 2003, 2008) and to choose life-prolonging treatment that, if of benefit to them, will sustain life. They are equally entitled to comprehensive packages of care to support their needs. Pfund (2007) discusses the availability of comprehensive local services to support technology-dependent children at home – that with appropriate implementation of the long-term ventilation guidelines (DH 2005a) and the Long term ventilation (LTV) pathway it is possible to provide effective care.

=== **ACTIVITY** ===

Consider the advances in medical technology and the increasing number of children being offered long-term ventilation. What are the ethical issues raised by this for health and social care delivery, the child and family?

End-of-life decisions

End-of-life decisions can be challenging and controversial (end-of- life care is discussed in chapter Chapter 9). Children with life-threatening conditions are now living longer (e.g.for example, those with conditions such as cystic fibrosis and Duchennes muscular dystrophy) when beforehand previously their conditions would have resulted in an earlier death. Advancing technology makes possible life- sustaining treatments in cases that were previously regarded as hopeless (RCPCH 2004). The consequence of this is that boundaries between basic care and treatment can become blurred, and decisions regarding life-prolonging treatment more difficult.

Two key concepts underpinning end–of-life decisions exist, being basic care and life-prolonging treatment.

Basic care

This is classed as care and procedures that are solely delivered to provide comfort to the child including warmth, shelter, hygiene measures, oral nutrition and hydration, and the provision of medication to relieve pain and suffering.

Life-prolonging treatment

This refers to all treatments or procedures that have the potential to postpone the patient's death, and includes cardiopulmonary resuscitation, artificial ventilation, specialized treatments such as chemotherapy, dialysis and antibiotics when given for a potentially life-threatening infection, artificial nutrition and hydration (BMA 2007).

Significant discussion has focused on withholding or withdrawing treatment, including artificial nutrition and hydration and cardiopulmonary resuscitation.

Withdrawing and withholding treatment

Decisions surrounding withholding and withdrawing treatment for children are never easy, yet in palliative care practice we have to decide whether to start, continue or stop treatment. Assumptions in health care would suggest that if life-prolonging treatment for children was to be beneficial then most families would want it. However, there are times when treatment fails to be of benefit, or the risk and consequences outweigh the benefits and it is considered appropriate to withhold or withdraw treatment.

Such decisions can cause tension and conflict, and there has been considerable discussion in the media and literature surrounding a number of cases with regard to care and treatment of adults (*Pretty* v. *The United Kingdom* 2002), young people (*Airedale NHS Trust* v. *Bland* 1993), and children (*Glass* v. *The United Kingdom* 2004, *Portsmouth NHS Trust* v. *Wyatt* 2005). Consideration of the legal and ethical aspects underpinning the withholding and withdrawal of treatment has resulted in some key guidelines and recommendations for practice.

Legal guidelines

▪ In law, there is no distinction between the withdrawal or withholding of life-prolonging treatment.

1. The 'brain dead' child – where two doctors have agreed brain stem death, further treatment is deemed futile and the withdrawal of current treatment is appropriate.
2. The 'permanent vegetative state' – for a child who is reliant on others for all care and does not respond or relate with the world as a result of trauma or hypoxia, withdrawal or withholding treatment may be appropriate.
3. The 'no chance' situation – the child has such severe disease that life-prolonging treatment simply delays death without any benefit. Treatment to sustain life is inappropriate.
4. The 'no purpose' situation – the child may be able to survive with life-prolonging treatment, the degree of physical or mental impairment is so great that it is unreasonable to expect the child to bear it.
5. The 'unbearable' situation – the child and/or family feel that, in the face of progressive illness, further treatment is more than they can bear and choose to have a particular treatment withdrawn. This may be irrespective of medical opinion that such treatment may be of some benefit.

Figure 4.4   Five situations where it may be ethical and legal to consider the withdrawal or withholding of life- sustaining treatment.

Source: RCPCH (2004).

- It is acceptable to withdraw life- prolonging treatment when the quality of life is such that there is no benefit to the child, or the treatment is deemed to be intolerable.

- All decisions to withdraw or withhold treatment should be carried out within the legal context of the child's rights, including the process for consent.

- If there is any disagreement that is unresolved, then the courts should be consulted legal advice can be obtained from the hospital management legal adviser, or from the Children and Family Court Advisory and Support Service.

Figure 4.4 lists five situations where it may be ethical and legal to consider withholding or withdrawing life-sustaining treatment.

It is recommended that if the criteria do not fit the situation, then life-prolonging treatment may be in the child's best interests, and that the decision should always be considered within the overall context of care.

KEY POINT

Legally, there is no difference between withdrawing or withholding life-prolonging treatment; however, emotionally, parents and health care professionals find it difficult to withdraw treatment.

Artificial nutrition and hydration

Artificial nutrition and hydration refers to the techniques for providing nutrition and hydration that are used to bypass an inability to swallow (dysphagia) (BMA 2007). When children have difficulty with swallowing and are unable to take oral fluids and nutrition, in particular those children with a neurodegenerative or neuromuscular condition, it may be appropriate to offer artificial nutrition and hydration.

Despite being common practice in many areas of children's palliative care, the delivery of artificial nutrition and hydration continues to attract wide-spread debate. The ethical discussion centres on whether artificial nutrition and hydration is a legal right, and the issues of withholding and withdrawing artificial nutrition and hydration.

The tension around artificial nutrition and hydration emerges because nutrition and hydration are acknowledged as basic care, which should always be provided; however, methods to provide artificial nutrition and hydration are regarded as medical treatment. Despite arguments to suggest a difference between the insertion of a tube and the delivery of nutrition via the tube, there is no distinction in law. This was a central question in the case of Tony Bland (1993) and is now established as common law (BMA 2007). In certain situations, it is therefore appropriate to consider the withdrawal of artificial nutrition and hydration. This should be done sensitively with full agreement from parents and in line with recommended principles and guidelines (see Figure 4.4, above). In particular, it is advised to get a second opinion when death is not imminent.

The need to balance the care of children regarding the withholding or withdrawing of artificial nutrition and hydration reflects a number of points highlighted in the previous section. Understanding the needs of the child and family, the child's best interests and his or her quality of life are essential. Evidence-based practice and clinical judgement will assist in promoting the best possible outcome.

CLINICAL FOCUS

Following a complicated delivery, resulting in birth asphyxia, Rebecca is diagnosed with severe and irreversible brain damage. Despite repeated attempts and coaxing, at three days old she is unable to suck or swallow. Her parents are keen not to further their baby's suffering and do not want a naso-gastric tube to be inserted for nutrition and hydration. However, there is tension among professionals caring for the baby. Some believe Rebecca's parents have a right to decide for their baby, while others raise questions regarding the best interests of Rebecca and argue that a naso-gastric tube should be inserted to maintain nutrition and hydration.

APPLICATION IN PRACTICE

Ethical issues explored

■ A multi-professional case conference outlining the medical background and presenting all options of treatment and care, including the short- and long- term consequences for the child and family need to be discussed.

- The best interests of the baby, and the rights and choices of the parents must be addressed.

- Current evidence regarding the delivery of nutrition and hydration for severely ill neonates, and care at the end of life, should be taken in to consideration.

- Guidelines on withholding and withdrawing treatment should be applied.

- A sensitive, ethical approach addressing principles and frameworks of ethical practice will help to achieve the best possible outcome for the child and family.

Cardiopulmonary resuscitation

Cardiopulmonary resuscitation (CPR) can be attempted on any person, child or adult, when cardiac or respiratory functions cease. A few patients will make a full recovery, some recover but have a number of health problems, but in most cases, restarting the heart and breathing, despite the best efforts of those involved, is unsuccessful.

For patients in poor health and those with serious conditions it is known to have a low success rate (BMA/RC/RCN 2001).

Advanced technology and life-prolonging treatments have extended the lives of children and young people, resulting in more families than before, choosing CPR as a life-prolonging treatment. But discussions regarding CPR raise sensitive and difficult issues for the family in particular around the best interests and quality of life. To achieve the best possible outcome, the views of the family and the medical and nursing team immediately involved in the child's care are valuable in coming to a decision. Ideally, discussions about resuscitation should be addressed in advance with the child (if appropriate) and family in a supportive relationship (RCPCH and RCN 2007). The meaning of cardiopulmonary resuscitation and an understanding of the process and consequences should be fully explored. In addition, discussions should involve other aspects of end-of-life care.

The values, wishes and illness experience of the child and family will help to determine the most appropriate action with regard to any resuscitation attempt, and when it is appropriate to make an advance decision *not* to attempt CPR. It is also important to assess the clinical situation and be guided by legal and local policy.

When discussing the appropriateness of cardiopulmonary resuscitation, an open and honest dialogue should take place, and the following issues (adapted from RCPCH and RCN 2007) should be considered:

- The severity and type of illness and disability of the child.

- The possible prognosis.

- Is CPR likely to restart the child's heart and breathing?

- Would restarting the child's heart and breathing provide any benefit – is it in their best interests?

■ The expected benefits weighed against the potential burdens and risks of the resuscitation process – quality of life following CPR.

■ The child's own wishes if he or she is able to share his/her views and wishes.

■ The wishes of the parents/guardians.

Any decision should be based on the best available evidence and information, and consensus within the team. All decisions should be shared and all details of the discussion documented.

Sanctity of life

The concept of sanctity of life holds the intrinsic value of being alive. It is understood not in terms of life as an absolute good, but that life must never be taken intentionally. Some people believe that life should be sustained at all costs, no matter what the quality, and that life-prolonging treatment provides a benefit despite any other factors.

Consequently, it can be challenging working within a diverse team who share multiple beliefs and perspectives of end-of-life care.

KEY POINT

When working within an interdisciplinary team dealing with end-of-life decisions, all values and beliefs should be respected, and sensitive support and supervision offered.

Euthanasia

In the past, the concept of euthanasia was understood to mean a good or easy death. Contemporary understanding describes euthanasia as the deliberate ending of life. Currently within the UK, active euthanasia is illegal for children and adults. However, for some, euthanasia is considered as acceptable practice while others believe it should never occur. Ongoing national and international debate may see changes to the law (see the section Physician-assisted suicide, below).

In relation to withdrawal of treatment, the Royal College of Paediatrics and Child Health (RCPCH 2004) emphasize that the courts do not see the withdrawal of life-sustaining treatment in appropriate circumstances as active killing (active euthanasia). It is also indicated that if withdrawal of treatment – for example, ventilatory support – does not lead to death, then euthanasia is not appropriate. If the child survives, even though badly disabled, he or she should be respected and cared for appropriately (RCPCH 2004).

Physician-assisted suicide

Physician-assisted suicide is the result of a deliberate medical act or omission taken by a doctor that shortens the life (hastens the death) of a patient. Current debate

---

Definitions of euthanasia

▪ Euthanasia – Literally translated, means 'good death'. A deliberate act or omission that shortens the life (hastens the death) of a person.

▪ Active euthanasia – The purposeful shortening of life through active or direct assistance.

▪ Passive euthanasia – The purposeful omission (by withdrawing or withholding) of life-sustaining measures.

▪ Voluntary euthanasia – The freely-given consent of the individual to his/her death.

▪ Involuntary – purposeful shortening of life without the individual's consent

▪ Nonvoluntary – When a life is taken when it is impossible to ask for an individual's consent e.g. incompetent or unconscious persons

---

Figure 4.5 Definitions of euthanasia

and interest is driven by Lord Joffe's Assisted Dying Bill (House of Lords 2005) advocating the rights of the individual who is suffering unbearably as a result of a life- threatening illness, to seek medical assistance to die at his or her own considered and persistent request.

The arguments and questions arising from the bill to legalize physician-assisted suicide have affected both children requiring palliative care and those with complex needs. Questions and fears around where the line would be drawn, the burden of care, the trust of the health care profession, and pressure on relatives to end life because of the impact of cost and resources have all been debated (Finlay *et al.* 2005).

The debate surrounding euthanasia and assisted dying will continue to attract public awareness and debate. Increasing attention will be given to the rights and best interests of the child in relation to euthanasia and assisted suicide. Health care professionals will need to be prepared to enter into such discussions.

Advance directives (living wills)

An advance directive (or living will) is a written or verbal statement made by an individual, and this can be a child. It is made at a time when the individual has the capacity to decide, and states the person's wishes regarding the acceptance or refusal of care, treatment and management of their illness.

Advance decisions for care and refusal of treatment are now also legally recognized for adults within the Mental Capacity Act (DH, 2005b).

Advance directives for children, although not acknowledged by law, give the child a voice and reflect government recommendations to ensure that the views of the child, particularly with regard to their preferred place of care (DH 2008). While in the United Kingdom advance directives for children are not legally accepted, many children are capable of providing guidance about their wishes for care, and health care professionals would be morally obliged to take such wishes into account (Friebert 2004). Discussion around their creation can often facilitate dialogue about end–of–life care that can inform the health care team.

Other ethical issues related to children's palliative care

Organ transplantation and tissue retention

Because of the nature of childhood conditions seen at the end of life, discussion surrounding organ transplantation at the time of death is not often raised. However, some families may gain great comfort in being able to consider organ transplantation, and part of the duty of care is to respect their wishes. With developing technology and controlled withdrawal of treatment, organ transplantation and tissue donation is possible, and if appropriate it should be facilitated. Anxiety among families has been created as a result of media attention surrounding events at Alder Hey and the subsequent Redfern Report (2001), so families should be fully informed of the process (McNeilly and Price, 2008) and information provided regarding how organs and tissues are to be used is essential.

Organ donation

As medicine and treatments advance, increasing attention is given to children, as donors, in the treatment of life- threatening conditions. Holm (2004) states that the issues around children, as donors, are by far the most difficult of ethical debates. It is argued from a number of perspectives. Crouth and Elliot (1999) raise the question for parents of allowing the interests of one child to be risked for the sake of another. Central to this debate is the interests of the child donor whose sibling will die without an organ transplant. However, Jansen (2004) argues that children, as donors, cannot be addressed simply by applying the principle of the best interests of either child. She claims that due weight should also be given to the interests of the family and the intimate relationships that families make possible. These debates will long continue within the professional and public field, and it is likely that limited common ground will be found. It is essential, as stated throughout this book, that sensitive, meaningful communication should take place to reach the best possible outcome that includes the whole family.

Genetic testing

Pre-natal genetic testing is becoming widely used in health care, and extends the ethical debate in society as to the appropriateness of genetic testing. However, for parents of a child with a life-threatening condition, testing can detect genetic abnormalities that provide information about the health of the foetus. For some families, the desire for this information can support decision-making when they already have a child or relative with a known condition.

In the United Kingdom, children under 18 are not considered to be mature enough to make fully informed decisions regarding genetic testing. Guidelines suggest that once a child reaches adulthood they will be able to decide for themselves (Clinical Genetic Society 1994) However, for some children and families there may be situations where genetic testing is beneficial: to gain knowledge of carrier status or specific testing for late-onset disorders, for example. Savulescu (2001) raises arguments both for and against genetic testing in children, and recognizes that this may be a challenging decision for both the child and the family. Early testing may help in psychological adjustment and resolve uncertainty, but it may also disturb family dynamics and create a sense of guilt for parents if a child tests positive for a condition or is a carrier (Savulescu 2001).

These challenges have been highlighted by the Department of Health in their report addressing the future of genetics within the NHS (DH 2003). Such development requires a comprehensive support programme for children and families surrounding the long-term implications following genetic testing, for which paediatric nurses require specific training.

Conclusion

Ethics is central to all areas of children's palliative care, and sensitive decision-making practice is key to achieving effective and positive choices for children and families. This chapter has addressed the ethical dimensions of children's palliative care and highlighted some of the key ethical challenges for practitioners.

Advances in medical technology that widen the choices and scope of treatment have contributed to an increase in the number of ethical debates in children's palliative care practice. As technology continues to develop, these ethical issues are likely to increase further in number and complexity. The dilemmas of consent, withdrawal of treatment and growing attention being paid to children as organ donors are some of the issues that can create tension and conflict among healthcare professionals and parents. However, by promoting a culture of open communication, and using an ethical approach that encompasses the child and family context, and acknowledges individual values and relationships, can help in the decision-making process. Such an approach will meet the needs of children and their families more effectively, providing support for them throughout the illness journey.

Key resources

British Medical Association (2007) *Withholding and Withdrawing Life-prolonging medical Treatment. Guidance for decision making.* London: British Medical Journal Books.

RCPCH (Royal College of Paediatrics and Child Health) (2004) *Withholding or Withdrawing Life Sustaining Treatment in Children. A Framework for Practice*, 2nd edn. London: RCPCH.

RCPCH and RCN (Royal College of Paediatrics and Child Health and Royal College of Nursing) (2007) *A Joint Statement. Decisions Relating to Cardiopulmonary Resuscitation.* London: RCPCH.

CHAPTER SUMMARY

▪ The challenges for ethics in children's palliative care are wide and diverse.

▪ An ethical approach to decision-making must take into account the contextual elements of children's palliative care practice.

▪ A feminist and situated ethical approach, in addition to understanding ethical principles, is a valuable dimension to the decision-making process.

▪ Attention to the child's rights and best interests are integral in all aspects of palliative care practice.

▪ It is important to promote and foster a culture of honest and sensitive communication where ethical dilemmas can be openly discussed.

▪ The withholding and withdrawing of treatment may be appropriate given certain situations – the RCPCH describes five situations where this may be appropriate.

▪ Artificial nutrition and hydration are regarded by the law as medical treatment, and in appropriate circumstances may be withdrawn.

▪ Any decision at the end of life should be based on best available evidence and information, the best interests of the child within the family context and a shared responsibility with the team.

References

Addington-Hall, J. (2002) Research sensitivities to palliative care patients. *European Journal of Cancer Care* **11**: 220–4.

Airedale NHS Trust v. *Bland* (1993) 1 A11 ER 821.

Alderson, P. (1992) In the genes or in the stars? Children's competence to consent. *Journal of Medical Ethics*. **18**: 119–24.

Alderson, P. (1995) *Listening to Children: Children, Ethics and Social Research*. London: Barnardo's.

Alderson, P. (2005) Complications with consent. *Bulletin of Medical Ethics* **210**: 15–19.

Alderson, P. and Montgomery, J. (1996) *Health Care Choices: Making Decisions with Children*. London: Institute for Public Policy Research.

Ashcroft, R. E. (2007) Preface. In Ashcroft, R. E., Dawson, A., Draper, H. and McMillan, J. R. (eds) *Principles of Health Care Ethics*, 2nd edn. Chichester: John Wiley.

Baston, J. (2008) Healthcare decisions: a review of children's involvement. *Paediatric Nursing* **20**(3): 24–6.

Beauchamp, T. and Childress, J. (2001) *Principles of Biomedical Ethics*, 5th edn. Oxford: Oxford University Press.

British Medical Association (2001) *Consent, Rights and Choices in Health Care for Children and Young People*. London: British Medical Journal Books.

British Medical Association (2007) *Withholding and Withdrawing Life-prolonging medical Treatment. Guidance for decision making*. London: British Medical Journal Books.

British Medical Association (2008) *Parental Responsibility*. Available at: www.bma.org.uk/ap.nsf/Content/Parental; accessed January 2008.

British Medical Association, the Resuscitation Council and Royal College of Nursing (2001) *A Joint Statement: Decisions Relating to Cardiopulmonary Resuscitation*. London: BMA/RCN.

Broome, M. (1999) Consent (assent) for research with pediatric patients. *Seminar of Oncology Nursing.* **15**: 96–103.

Burns, J. (2003) Research in children. *Critical Care Medicine* **31**(3): S131-S136.

Casarett, D. (2005) Ethical considerations in end-of-life care and research. *Journal of Palliative Medicine* **8**: S148-S160.

Northern Ireland Assembly (1995) *Children (Northern Ireland) Order.* Belfast: HMSO.

Clinical Genetics Society, The (1994) *What is Clinical Genetics?* Available at: www.clingensoc.org; accessed January 2008.

Crouth, R. A. and Elliot, C. (1999) Moral agency and the case of living related organ transplantation. *Cambridge Quarterly Health Care Ethics* **8**: 275–87.

DH (Department of Health) (1969) *The Family Law Reform Act.* DH. London: Department of Health.

DH (Department of Health) (1989) *The Children Act.* London: Department of Health.

DH (Department of Health) (2000) *The Human Rights Act.* London: Department of Health.

DH (Department of Health) (2003) *Every Child Matters.* London: Department of Health.

DH (Department of Health) (2004a) *The Children Act.* London: Department of Health.

DH (Department of Health) (2004b) *The National Service Framework for Children, Young People and Maternity Services.* London: Department of Health.

DH (Department of Health) (2005a) *National Service Framework for Children and Young People and Maternity Services: Long Term Ventilation.* London: Department of Health.

DH (Department of Health) (2005b) *The Mental Capacity Act.* London: Department of Health.

DH (Department of Health) (2008) *Better Care: Better Lives.* London: Department of Health. Available at: www2.ohchr.org/english/law/disabilities-convention.htm.

Dimond, B. (2002) *Legal Aspects of Nursing,* (3rd edn). Harlow: Longman.

Edwards, R. and Mauthner, M. (2002) Ethics and feminist research: theory and practice. In Mauthner, M., Birch, M., Jessop, J. and Miller, T. *Ethics in Qualitative Research.* London: Sage.

Eiser, C. (1990) *Chronic Childhood Disease: An Introduction to Psychological Theory and Research.* Cambridge: Cambridge University Press.

Fajerman, J., Treseder, P. and Connor, J. (2004) *Children are Service Users Too. A Guide to Consulting Children and Young People.* London: Save the Children.

Feudtner, C. (2007) Collaborative communication in pediatric palliative care: a foundation for problem solving and decision-making. *Pediatric Clinics of North America* **54**(5): 583–607.

Finlay, I. G., Wheatley, V.J. and Izdebski, C. (2005) The House of Lords Select Committee on Assisted Dying for the Terminally Ill Bill: implications for specialist palliative care. *Palliative Medicine* **19**: 444–53.

Foster, C. (2001) *The Ethics of Medical Research on Humans.* Cambridge: Cambridge University Press.

Friebert, S. (2004) *Health Care Decision-making in Pediatric Palliative Care. The National Alliance for Children with Life Threatening Conditions.* Available at: www.nacwltc.org; accessed March 2004.

Friedman Ross, L. (ed.) (2001) *Children, Families and Health Care Decision Making.* Oxford: Clarendon Press.

Gibson, C. (1993) Underpinnings of ethical reasoning in nursing. *Journal of Advanced Nursing* **18**: 2003–7.

Gillick v. *West Norfolk & Wisbech AHA & DHSS* (1983) 3, WLR (QBD).

Gillick v. *West Norfolk & Wisbech AHA & DHSS* (1985) 3, WLR (HL).

Glass v. *The United Kingdom* (2004) 1 FLR 1019.

Heaton, J., Noyes, J., Sloper, P. and Shah, R. (2003) Technology dependent children and family life. *Research Works, 2003–02,* York: University of York, Social Policy Research Unit.

Hendrick, J. (2000) *Law and Ethics in Nursing and Health Care.* Cheltenham: Stanley Thornes.

Higgs, R. (2007) Truth telling, lying and the doctor–patient relationship. In Ashcroft, R. E., Dawson, A., Draper, H. and McMillan, J. R. (eds) *Principles of Health Care Ethics,* 2nd edn. Chichester: John Wiley.

Hinds, P. S., Oakes, L., Furman, W. *et al.* (1997) Decision making by parents and healthcare professionals when considering continued care for paediatric patients with cancer. *Oncology Nursing Forum.* **24**(9): 1523–8.

Hinds, P. S., Oakes, L., Furman, W. *et al.* (2001) End-of-life decision making by adolescents, parents and healthcare providers in pediatric oncology. *Cancer Nursing* **24**(2): 122–36.

Holm, S. (2004) The child as organ and tissue donor: discussions in the Danish Council of Ethics. *Cambridge Quarterly Health Care Ethics* **13**: 156–60.

Hope, T., Savulescu, J. and Hendrick, J. (2003) *Medical Ethics and Law. The Core Curriculum.* London: Churchill Livingstone.

House of Lords (2005) Assisted Dying for the Terminally Ill Bill. London: The Stationery Office.

Jansen, L. A. (2004) Child organ donation, family autonomy and intimate attachments. *Cambridge Quarterly Health Care Ethics* **13**: 133–42.

Jardine, E., O'Toole, M., Payton, J. Y. and Wallis, C. (1999) Current status of long term ventilation of children in the United Kingdom: questionnaire survey. *British Medical Journal* **318**: 295–9.

Leikin, S. (1993) Minor's assent, consent, or dissent to medical research. *Institutional Review Board* **15**(2): 1–7.

Lowden, J. (2002) Children's rights: a decade of dispute. *Journal of Advanced Nursing* **317**(1): 100–7.

McConnell, Y., Frager, G. and Levetown, M. (2004) Decision making in pediatric palliative care. In Carter, S. and Levetown, M. (eds) *Palliative Care for Infants, Children and Adolescents. A Practical Handbook.* Baltimore, MD: Johns Hopkins University Press.

McNeilly , P. and Price, J. (2008) Care of the child after death. In Kelsey, J. and McEwing, G. (eds) *Clinical Skills in Child Health Practice.* Oxford: Elsevier Press.

Morrow, V. and Richards, M. (1996) The ethics of social research with children. An overview. *Children and Society* **10**: 90–105.

National Children's Bureau (NCB) (2008) *Participation and Children's Rights.* Available at: www.ncb.org.uk; accessed March 2008.

Pfund, R. (2007) *Palliative care nursing of children and young people.* Oxford: Radcliffe Publishing.

Portsmouth NHS Trust v. *Wyatt* (2005) 1 FLR 21.

Pretty v. *The United Kingdom* (2002) 2 FLR 45.

Randall, F. and Downie, R. (1999) *Palliative Care Ethics,* (2nd edn) Oxford: Oxford University Press.

Redfern, M. (2001) *The Report of the Royal Liverpool Inquiry.* London: HMSO. Available at: www.rlcinquiry.org.uk

RCN (Royal College of Nursing) (2006) Informed consent in health and social care research: RCN guidance for nurses. Available at: *www.rcn.org.uk*; accessed June 2006.

RCPCH (Royal College of Paediatrics and Child Health) (2004) *Withholding or Withdrawing Life Sustaining Treatment in Children. A Framework for Practice,* 2nd edn. London: RCPCH.

RCPCH and RCN (Royal College of Paediatrics and Child Health and Royal College of Nursing) (2007) *A Joint Statement. Decisions Relating to Cardiopulmonary Resuscitation.* London: RCPCH.

Save the Children (2008) Research and resources. Available at: www.savethechildren.org.uk; accessed March 2008.

Savulescu, J. (2001) Predictive genetic testing in children. *Medical Journal of Australia* **175**: 379–81.

Scottish Government (1995) *Children (Scotland) Act.* London: HMSO.

Tuckett, A. (2004) Truth-telling in clinical practice and the arguments for and against: a review of the literature. *Nursing Ethics* **11**(5): 500–13.

Children (Northern Ireland) Order (1995) Belfast: HMSO.

United Nations (1989) *The United Nations Convention on the Rights of The Child.* Available at: www.unhchr.ch; accessed July 2007.

United Nations (2007) *Convention on the Rights of Persons with Disabilities.* Available at www2.ohchr.org/english/law/disabilities-convention.htm

Walker, M. (1998) *Moral Understandings: A Feminist Study in Ethics*. New York: Routledge.

Wheeler, R. (2006) Gillick or Fraser? A plea for consistency over competency in children. *British Medical Journal* **332**: 807.

Woods. M. (2001) Balancing rights and duties in 'life and death' decision making involving children: a role for nurses. *Nursing Ethics* **8**(5): 397–408.

Meeting the Spiritual Needs of Children and Families

Wilfred McSherry and Sue Jolley

Introduction

The diagnosis of a life-threatening or life-limiting illness can be devastating for all concerned. Life is often turned upside down and the resulting anxiety and uncertainty can have a catastrophic impact on the patient, and their family and friends. In such situations, individuals may start to question the very meaning and purpose of life, challenging long-held beliefs and values in an attempt to make sense of their situation and restore some order to the chaos they may be encountering (NICE 2004). These situations are traumatic for anyone, but for children they are compounded by other factors, such as the inability to make sense of the world around them and a lack of language to express innermost fears and concerns (McSherry and Smith 2007). Often these factors are combined with imaginary, unsubstantiated uncertainties stemming from an immature understanding of life and death. Therefore, the resulting care must take into consideration the developmental stage of the child so they may engage with and feel comfortable with the caring process.

Palliative care services are prepared to address the physical, psychological and social needs of patients, but the area of spirituality and the provision of spiritual care still prove to be stumbling blocks for many health care professionals. This may be for a number of reasons, such as misconceptions associated with spirituality and spiritual care; fear of mismanagement; or individuals' unease and reservations regarding the concepts. Again, all these issues are exacerbated when caring for children with palliative care needs. This chapter introduces practitioners to the concept of spirituality and explores the implications of dealing with children's and families' spiritual needs within palliative care services.

Drivers for spiritual care

There are numerous political and professional drivers that are advocating and promoting the inclusion of spirituality within the delivery of holistic and palliative care. A good starting point would be to explore the World Health Organization's definition of palliative care for children (WHO 2008: 1): 'Palliative care for children is the active total care of the child's body, mind and spirit, and also involves giving support to the family.' Within this definition, explicit reference to the spiritual dimension is made. There is an emphasis on treating all dimensions of the child. Guidelines for the delivery of religious and spiritual care have been developed in the United Kingdom (Scottish Executive Health Department 2002, DH 2003, NICE 2004). These guidelines have had a dramatic impact on the organization and delivery of religious and spiritual care in Scotland. However, in England, Wales and Northern Ireland, there has been less of an impact, and this area is still being developed. NICE (2004) raises the profile of spiritual care when they include this as an integral part of supportive palliative care. The Nursing and Midwifery Council (2004) have identified that pre-registration nursing students should achieve competency in providing holistic care. These political and professional drivers may have inadvertently increased health care professionals' awareness of the need to treat all patients, both adults and children, holistically. Importantly, the principles and practices outlined in such guidance need to be transferred into paediatric or children's palliative care services.

 ACTIVITY

Spend several minutes reflecting on your understanding of the word 'spirituality'.

Write down any thoughts, words, feelings, images that come into your mind as you think about the word.

Defining spirituality

The concept of spirituality is now firmly established as an integral and fundamental component within nursing and health care practice. This may be in part a result of the drive for holistic care. However, there seem to be few articles or studies exploring the spiritual needs of children needing palliative care, and those of their families. Yet there is an emerging literature base related to the spiritual needs of children generally within nursing, and primary and secondary education (Anderson and Steen 1995, Steen and Anderson 1995, Seden 1998, Kenny 1999, Pfund 2000, Smith and McSherry 2004, Kenny and Ashley 2005, McSherry and Smith 2007). The authors are acutely aware of the danger of imposing or overgeneralizing adult principles of spirituality on children, and indeed this is not being advocated. Nevertheless, in light of the limited evidence base focusing on children's spirituality, the adult literature provides a useful framework from which to begin discussion and exploration of the concepts within the context of children.

An important message from the published literature is that there is no real consensus or authoritative definition of what constitutes spirituality (Narayanasamy 2001). Your own reflections while carrying out the Activity (on page 89) might have revealed that you have not given any real thought to the word, or indeed have no real understanding of what constitutes spirituality. Alternatively, you might have identified several words or feelings that reflect and capture your understanding. Your reflections may have revealed spirituality to be:

- Something at the centre of your being.

- Inner peace, inner strength.

- Personal beliefs, attitudes.

- Connectedness to nature or a supreme being.

- A religious belief.

- Belief in God.

- Love and happiness.

One of the most frequently used definitions of spirituality in the health care literature is the one provided by Murray and Zentner (1989: 259). According to these authors, spirituality is:

> A Quality that goes beyond religious affiliation, that strives for inspirations, reverence, awe, meaning and purpose, even in those who do not believe in any good. The spiritual dimension tries to be in harmony with the universe, and strives for answers about the infinite, and comes into focus when the person faces emotional stress, physical illness or death.

This definition reveals that spirituality is complex and multifaceted, in that it can be viewed in many different ways. It implies that spirituality is universal, deeply personal and individual. It applies to all people: those with a religious belief, and those who hold none. Spirituality is intricately linked with existentialism; that is, the need to find meaning, purpose and fulfilment in life. This definition of spirituality did not emerge out of any empirical study, and a problem with it is that it is most definitely written with adults in mind. The language used, and the many descriptions provided, will undoubtedly be unfamiliar for many children.

Therefore, a more pragmatic and less intellectual definition of spirituality and a model of spiritual care need to be developed and used that capture the spirit of the child. Children's spirituality is expressed and experienced more at an emotional level. Some children cannot articulate concepts and feelings, nor may they possess the ability to rationalize or reflect on matters of life, existence and death because of their age, or level of social and intellectual development. This ability may also have been impaired as a result of the nature of their illness, disorder or disease, but it does not mean that the concept of spirituality is obsolete or redundant. On the contrary, just because children may not articulate or identify with the concepts that adults use, it does not mean that they are unable to experience or express themselves at a spiritual level. All children of whatever age can sense goodness, love, happiness, joy and pain, and this may be expressed through a laugh, a smile, or even verbally. It is as more about connections with people, nature and transcendence than about intellectualizing and rationalizing. This point is crucial when caring for the spiritual needs of children within the context of palliative care. For those caring for such children and their families, it is not so much about what we say, but more about how we do things and the qualities that we, as health care professionals, display when providing care. Turner (1996) indicates that spiritual care is about being with patients as opposed to doing things to them. Spiritual care, if this exists, is hidden and revealed in the human elements of the caring and therapeutic process.

KEY POINT

There is no authoritative definition of what constitutes spirituality (Narayanasamy 2001).

Imperative questions

Irrespective of how we view or define spirituality, there are a number of important questions that health care professionals must ask, especially when caring for children within palliative care:

- What is spirituality, and how does this relate or manifest itself when caring for children requiring palliative care?

- Are health care professionals aware of how spirituality may be expressed by children with palliative care needs?

- Are we more concerned with a medical approach to care?

These questions are important because they will dictate whether this area is addressed within practice.

Religion and spirituality

One cannot look at the concept of spirituality without acknowledging the importance of religion. For some children and their families, religious belief, practices and customs, with associated teachings and doctrines, will be fundamental to their spirituality and lives. Any attempt to divorce the religious and theistic (idea of God or a deity) from spirituality is misguided and unwarranted within health care practice. There seems to be a decline in formal religious practice within the United Kingdom, but one cannot make generalizations and assume that religion is no longer important. For some children, their spirituality will be intricately interwoven with a religious belief. This belief may have been inherited or passed down to them from their parents, becoming an essential part of their life, identity and ancestry. This point is important, particularly now when health care

Table 5.1 Distinguishing the concepts of religion and spirituality

Religion	Spirituality
Community-focused	Individualistic
Observable, measurable, objective	Less visible and measurable, more subjective
Formal orthodox, organized	Less formal, orthodox, less systematic
Behavior orientated, outward practices	Emotionally orientated, inward directed
Authoritarian in terms of behavior	Not authoritarian, little accountability
Doctrine separating good from evil	Unifying, not doctrine orientated

Source: Koenig et al. (2001). Reproduced with the kind permission of Oxford University Press.

professionals are caring for children and families from diverse cultural, ethnic and religious backgrounds.

Koenig *et al.* (2001: 18) provide a useful table distinguishing the concepts of religion and spirituality (see Table 5.1). While this table highlights some of the important differences between these concepts, it is very rudimentary and not at all definitive.

It is not possible to discuss all the major world religions and their associated teachings, and the impact that these may have on caring for children within palliative care services. Many institutions and organizations now have resource guides or packs providing an overview of the main tenants of a particular religion and highlighting key doctrines, rituals and practice; for example, those associated with dietary requirements, or dress and modesty. These guides should never replace talking to individual children, parents and families about what they believe, and how their beliefs can be supported by staff. All people working with children in paediatric palliative care need awareness, education and information about the diverse customs and practices connected with the many world religions they might encounter (See Further Reading box below). By developing this awareness, health care professionals will be in a better position to offer culturally sensitive religious and spiritual care and avoid stereotypical assumptions and generalizations (Gilliat-Ray 2001).

═══════════════ **FURTHER READING** ═══════════════

For a more detailed discussion on the major world religions, the following titles are useful:

- Henley, A. and Schott, J. (1999) *Culture, Religion and Patient Care in a Multi-Ethnic Society*. London: Age Concern
- Neuberger, J. (2004) *Caring for Dying People of Different Faiths*, 3rd edn. Oxford: Radcliffe Publishing.

Models representing the spiritual dimension

No model will really capture or fully explain the spiritual dimension that resides within each individual child. It is beyond the scope of this chapter to provide such an explanation. However, what is required is some explanation or illustration of how spirituality may be located within each individual child, parent or family, to understand how spirituality may have an impact on the child's well-being. This type of explanation may assist practitioners working within paediatric palliative care services to look beyond the physical and medical domains. It must be borne in mind that a model is the views of one or two people as to how individuals are made, function and interact with the world. Therefore, models of spirituality or spiritual care represent a set of ideas, thoughts and, perhaps, a loose set of theories about how people's lives are constructed and how spirituality might influence and manifest itself within the caring relationship.

McSherry (2006; 52) describes spirituality in the terms of a football (see Figure 5.1), and other models may provide a similar explanation, such as a patchwork quilt. If the model of a football is applied to caring for children with palliative care needs, then the following points may be relevant:

- *Football* denotes the 'whole child' including their context, embracing family and friends.

- *Patches* are different dimensions of the child's being physical, psychological, social and spiritual. This includes other factors such as environmental ones.

- *Black patches* are aspects of life that health care professionals feel comfortable in addressing, such as physical and psychosocial needs. These areas of care are usually objective and tangible.

- *White patches* are areas of the child that are not so visible, less tangible but have a profound impact on the child, such as beliefs, values, creeds, cultural, religious and ethnic influences.

- *Thread* symbolizes the unifying force of spirituality, a force that integrates and permeates every dimension and aspect of life, whether children or adults are aware of this dimension within themselves or not.

- *Air* inflates the ball, providing it with shape and resilience. This is the life force. This force sustains the child and the family, enabling them to deal with situations both good and bad. It is this force that enables children to face the most difficult of situations courageously. When this force is extinguished, then the child ceases to exist and death occurs.

KEY POINT

Spirituality is thought to be universal, individual, personal and private. The concept applies to all children: those who have a religious belief and those who do not.

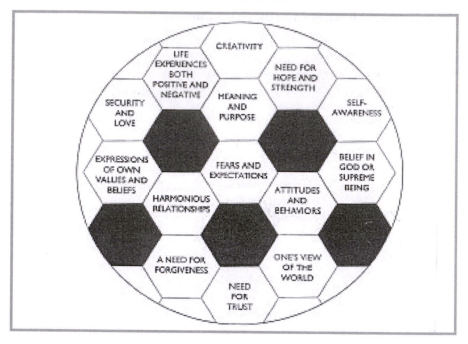

Figure 5.1 Spirituality as a football

Source: McSherry (2006: 52). Reproduced with the kind permission of Jessica Kingsley Publishers Ltd.

The spiritual needs of children

The logical progression and extension of the argument that everyone possesses spirituality is that everyone therefore has spiritual needs. With this point in mind, Table 5.2 presents nine spiritual needs that are considered central to every person irrespective of age and development.

=== **ACTIVITY** ===

Read through each of the spiritual needs identified in Table 5.2 and consider whether these have a meaning, significance and relevance to you. You may want to reflect on experiences encountered that would help you relate these to your own area of practice.

Spiritual assessment

Having briefly explored the concept of spiritual need, there is now a requirement to discuss how health care professionals and carers may assess or establish whether a child or his/her family has any need(s) in this area. It is not the intention of this chapter to provide a detailed discussion surrounding spiritual assessment. Spiritual assessment may be undertaken using different levels and forms, ranging from a general enquiry into a child's (family's) religious, cultural beliefs and practices. NICE (2004: 98), discussing spiritual support and services, state:

Table 5.2   Children's spiritual needs

Meaning and purpose
Children desire and need to explore the meaning of life and existence. Obviously, the level of exploration will be dependent upon age and stage of development. Such exploration will assist in generating their motivation or purpose, which will lead to a sense of fulfilment. This need to search is undertaken both when healthy and during times of illness.

Love and relationships
All children require intimacy and comfort derived from sharing love with others such as parents, siblings and friends. This is particularly important in the context of palliative care, where children can feel threatened, isolated and alone. In some situations they may feel deprived of the personal, intimate contact of parents. In order to develop socially and psychologically, children require security and love. These are all-important needs derived from personal contact and involvement with people, or contact with animals and creation.

Need for forgiveness
Parents will know that children can be very trying and frustrating. This can lead to a sense of anger and resentment, not only in the parent(s) but also in the child. Unresolved anger and guilt can lead to loss of physical, psychological, social and spiritual wellbeing, in both the parent and child. Therefore, in order to maintain a sense of peace, there is a need to try to resolve conflict speedily so that a resolution can be found, and forgiveness given if necessary, so that peace is restored.

Need for a source of hope and strength
Children are described by parents as the hope for the future, in terms of family and the world. Spiritually, children, by their very nature, inspire hope and are often a great source of strength to parents in the greatest adversity and the direst of circumstances. A child who is terminally ill can radiate such courage and resilience as they tolerate months of treatment. Consideration must be given to the child's personal beliefs, values and attitudes surrounding people and their future. For some children, strength and hope may be drawn from a religious perspective, such as the idea of heaven, or a place of peace; such beliefs will enable them to draw strength.

Creativity
Observing children at play is very inspiring because of their use of imagination and creativity. A simple cardboard box can be turned into a castle or a doll's house. Creativity is part of the child's natural world. By tapping into and harnessing this innate ability, one can help children to face the most harrowing of situations and experiences. Children and adults, by utilizing their creative forces such as by writing poetry or stories, or using art and music, enables them to express inner thoughts as well as a means of communication. Creativity can raise the child's awareness and enable the expression of hidden emotions and feelings.

Trust
Children require a sense of trust and stability in order to become well-adjusted citizens. If children are deprived of trust they may experience a sense of isolation and loneliness. Children encounter trust in a range of situations; within themselves, in their family and between friends. In today's climate, there is a growing concern because society or the world at large is overwhelming for many children, creating a sense of bewilderment and

uncertainty. Some children have lost hope and trust in a future and are sceptical of those in authority, such as politicians, teachers and even parents. Despite these concerns, trust is a prerequisite for establishing friendships and therapeutic relationships. Trust is fundamental to a child's existence and imperative for good communication. Trust leads to a sense of value, self-worth and acceptance by the self and others.

Maintain religious and spiritual practices

As children develop and mature, there may be certain religious or spiritual practices they have adopted or fashioned. These practices may originate from within a religious framework or be inherited from their parents, such as the need for daily prayer or attendance at church services or the synagogue, mosque or temple. However, some children may have no formal religious belief but may have grown spiritually through other activities such as attending a youth group or movement, participating in sports or expressing themselves creatively through other hobbies or pastimes. During periods of illness or hospitalization there will be a need to ensure that such religious or spiritual practices are maintained where possible. This may necessitate liaising with the Chaplaincy team and the child's own religious or spiritual leader.

Express one's own belief in God or a deity

An important dimension of spirituality for some children will be their belief in a God or supreme power or being. This may be a belief in a God who is creator of the world, as, for example, in the Judeo-Christian tradition. Dawkins (2006) cautions that children are too young to know whether they believe in a specific religion and that there is no such thing as a 'Muslim child' or a 'Catholic child', suggesting we should talk in terms of a child of Catholic parents. Yet children do adopt and often share the same belief system as their parents. Whether individuals agree with this point, religion and belief in a God may be an essential component of some children's lives. However, for some children they may have no conception of a God, supreme being or deity. Nevertheless, they may have a sense of 'something out there', an awareness of something greater than themselves, a sense of transcendence.

Ability to express one's own personal beliefs and values

In life there is a primary need for children to express and explore their own personal beliefs and values. As children develop and mature they may start to question long-established beliefs and values, often inherited from their parents. This questioning is normally associated with a desire for independence and personal autonomy. This may be evident in health care as children question treatment options. The inability to express one's own personal beliefs and values can lead to frustration and eventually hostility.

Source: Adapted from McSherry (2006: 56–7). Reproduced with the kind permission of Jessica Kingsley Publishers Ltd.

> Teams should ensure accurate and timely evaluation of spiritual issues is facilitated through a form of assessment based on recognition that spiritual needs are likely to change with time and circumstances. Assessment of spiritual needs does not have to be structured, but should include core elements such as exploring how people make sense of what happens to them.

While this is in relation to supporting patients with cancer, the principles could be applied to all people requiring palliative care, including children. Any form of spiritual assessment should be concerned with preserving the child's and the family's dignity and respect, and protecting the child's sense of worth and identity. Spiritual assessment should not be divisive, intrusive or offensive. There are many acronym-based assessment tools that may assist health care professionals to explore the spiritual dimension of care with children and families (Anandarajah and Hight 2001, Puchalski and Romer 2002). Again, these tools have been constructed with adults in mind, but with some modification they could be used within children's palliative care services. Before health care professionals rush ahead in constructing such tools, they may need to consider some of the ethical and practical implications linked to this area. McSherry and Ross (2002) provide a useful discussion of the different approaches to spiritual assessment and the ethical dilemmas practitioners might encounter.

Children's expressions of spiritual needs

Models of care often focus on the age of the child. However, developmental understanding and ability to express oneself is more important than age and physical ability when health professionals are attempting to facilitate spiritual communication. Adults may unknowingly impede expressions of spirituality in a child by trying to influence activities too much. Doka (1994, cited in Pfund 2000) supports this and suggests that the child should be encouraged to be involved in events as much as they wish without adult restriction – daily activities do not have to have a religious focus but should energize the child and family and assist in the spiritual journey. While it is recognized that all professionals working with children will understand the importance and role of play as a building block to communication, the emphasis in this chapter is on encouraging health care professionals to link 'play' more closely with spiritual development. Pfund (2000) suggests that there is little text available to address the difficulties in such provision of spiritual need and expression when working with children and their families. Table 5.3 may assist health care professionals in identifying how children express their spiritual selves at various developmental stages.

Spiritual care

Much of the care that is delivered within palliative care is focused on care management and ensuring that a child receives the best quality of physical care; families and carers rightly focus on the ability to say they did all they could; for example, that the child was always well dressed and not in discomfort. While no one would disregard such values – and indeed they are key elements of successful care delivery – it is important to consider the needs of the child to express his/her individuality and feelings/thoughts at the time. It is also important to acknowledge that spiritual expression is ever-changing; it is not sufficient merely to allow the child to do it once and then move on and never revisit that aspect of the child's care.

To a great extent, the activity associated with palliative care with children could be deemed distraction therapy. Activities are performed involving art work, pet therapy, music and sensory room space. The challenge is to ensure that

Table 5.3 Children's expressions of spiritual needs

Age	Examples of children's expressions of inner thoughts that may have a spiritual dimension	How these needs may be met in practice	Key developmental stages (Erikson 1963, Piaget 1952)
First year of life	Babies under one year express comfort and sadness with a combination of cries and calm behaviour. It is possible for those working closely with the baby to develop an understanding of the intensity of the cry to determine the 'problem'. Contentment is usually expressed by relaxed posture and interest in their world.	Touch, such as in the form of baby massage and the opportunity to feel safe when cuddled will provide positive connections with the baby, which may result in relaxation and a sense of peace. Use of musical toys to soothe and warm water to allow free movement may also elicit relaxation.	A sense of trust can develop during infancy in response to feeling comfort and having basic needs met. A tentative link has been made between the support parents provide an infant with and an ability to foster spiritual wellbeing.
Late infancy and toddlerhood	Ellie aged 2 years becomes very distressed and cries all day when left in the nursery while her mother visits her sibling in hospital. Ellie does not understand that her mother will be coming back and can only relate to the fact that she has gone.	Use of familiar stories and toys will enable security and inner peace. Routine is also important when considering the need to feel safe and relaxed within an environment and the company of others. Connections may be made with carers, by use of such strategies, which may facilitate expressions of self.	This is a time when young children will try to explore further their secure world. However, they are only willing to try new things on their own terms within the security of their main carer. If you remove the main carer, then the child's world loses its security blanket. Children at this age may take meanings very literally. In this example of the 2-year-old, it is possible to see that while the child is aware that her mother still exists, she has little understanding of when or if she will return.

Early school age	Mary, aged 5 years, was unusually difficult at school and would not co-operate with her friends as she would previously have done. The teacher was aware that Mary's father had recently undertaken a job abroad and would not be back for many weeks.	Routine and familiar objects remain very important to this age group. The need to express self is inhibited by lack of verbal language skills. Using paint, modelling clay and toys may enable the child to tell their story through the actions of their play.	At this age, the child experiences a challenging, widening social world where active, purposeful behaviour is needed to cope with these challenges. There may be a link between Mary's spiritual distress, fears and anxiety, which are being exhibited through disruptive behaviour.
Junior school years	Anita, aged 8, told the nurse that 'her brother had had the car accident because he was naughty at home last night. She was sure that he had caused the injury himself and was frightened in case she got ill because she had also been naughty at home yesterday'.	Utilizing stories may be useful at this age to allow the child to consider complex thoughts and see the world from the perspective of others. Discussions about cause and effect of illness may be possible and utilization of animal therapy may enable connections to be made between reality and the effects of care.	At this age, the child develops a sense of responsibility. Amy may be associating her brother's accident with wrong doing, and the consequential injury has become self-inflicted.
Middle school years	Ahmed, aged 11, told his teacher he was very happy today because he could walk to school but was sad because his friend would not be able to walk again due to falling off his horse and injuring his back. Ahmed was suddenly aware of how grateful he was for commonplace activity.	Discussions regarding how the child feels may be possible with the use of drawing to guide the conversation and assist the child to express his/her perspective. Considering how they themselves feel and the relationship they have with others may be enabled by children's inclusion in games and guided activities such as parachute play.	Children at this age are developing a sense of awareness of the needs of others and can incorporate their own life experience and relate the two, to draw conclusions about their own quality of life.

Table 5.3   Continued

| Adolescence | Alison was 16 when diagnosed with cancer. She found that she was unable to spend time with her friends because they were frightened to call her in case she wanted to talk about her illness. Alison became argumentative and disruptive at home and began to seek out new ways to gain attention – she began to smoke but also took out her old toys from the cupboard and placed them on her bed. | Adolescents are striving for independence but also require the security they had when they were smaller. Independent actions and activities, even when disruptive, may create a sense of achievement but the role of close contact with family and friends should not be forgotten to help facilitate self-expression. Use of complex language may be appropriate, but it may also be the case that the adolescent seeks to simplify and use language of the younger child because it is easier and enables expression of self. Return to familiar toys may surprise the adults around but shows a need for the world to remain constant. In such actions the adolescent may feel safe enough to express inner thoughts. | Adolescents are faced with many new experiences; independence as well as reliance on others. Alison needed her friends to call her, but those around her failed to identify the link between her behaviour and her lack of inner peace and wellbeing. |

Source: Adapted from McSherry and Smith (2007). Adapted and reproduced with the kind permission of *Paediatric Nursing*/ RCN Publishing Company.

the deliverers of care – whether health care professionals or family – are supported and encouraged to look beyond the involvement of the child and consider what he or she may be feeling and trying to 'say'. There is a need to look for small indicators of peace, contentment and individuality during activities.

Many activities, such as art work, are focused on 'decorating the room' or providing seasonal gifts to take home for the family – normal activities for children and no doubt much valued by the family. However, would it also be possible to include freedom of expression, such as paint-throwing, messy paint games, balloon popping or football kicking that might encourage a child to express deeply held thoughts that have no other means of release.

For many children in palliative care areas, the disease process takes many years, and much degeneration of physical and psychological function can occur during that time. Children who may have been able at one time to run wild and free may find themselves confined to wheelchairs with limited or impaired speech. While their mental understanding may remain intact, it is hard then for the child to let those around them know how they are feeling. Other children find that they have never had an opportunity to communicate with speech or movement, and the challenge for carers and family here is to understand how the child may express fear, anxiety, pain and pleasure. In these situations, carers become aware of familiar movements, facial expression and sounds that may enable an understanding of the child's inner self. It is then hard to develop further spiritual communication to enable the child to feel fulfilled and for the family to express their holistic needs.

=== **ACTIVITY** ===

Consider a child you may have cared for who has developed beyond the original expected level. Are family and staff pushing too hard to develop the child's progress further, or are they working at the level the child desires and, despite the child becoming tired and exhausted, allowing the child to play as freely as they wish without restraint.

Children's palliative care environments are increasingly providing care to children who were thought to have 'not long to live'. However, with the advancement of medicine, science and technology they are progressing beyond the wildest dreams of those who know them. This ability to maintain life against great odds may present health care professionals with a difficult challenge. Should they strive for further development and growth of the child, or acknowledge that this is still most likely to be limited and allow the child the freedom they deserve while it is possible? These difficult ethical and clinical dilemmas are explored in the following case study:

CLINICAL FOCUS

Fred is now 15 years old and was not expected to live beyond early childhood. He has cardiac disease and associated respiratory difficulties. He has become oxygen dependant and receives TPN nutrition for 16 hours per day. He also has moderate learning difficulties. Despite this, he is a lively young man who likes to engage with his peers, but is easily tired. In order to ensure he does not get too tired, which 'may affect his progress', the family restrict his activity to short periods during the day, have begun removing him from school on many occasions and are increasingly encouraging him to use a wheelchair for mobility.

Question 1: Is it possible that Fred's restricted mobility may affect his freedom to achieve spiritual fulfilment?

Question 2: Is it also possible that the family may require further support to enable them to come to terms with the potential deterioration of Fred and the importance of free expression and being oneself?

It would be wrong to present an impression here that the case study discussed in the Clinical Focus box above is in some way inappropriate care of the child. On the contrary, all involved are doing their best and the child is essentially happy, but the situation should be challenged because sometimes the spiritual needs of both family and child may be forgotten in such a focus on physical care. However, let us not forget that holism is also a form of spiritual management and, as Watson (2006) and Hull (1998) remind us, the child is not just the spirit but the physical as well. The Department of Health paper *Every Child Matters* (DH 2004) focuses entirely on physical needs and care. As a result, Watson (2006) would argue that children are not fully considered because spirituality is omitted. Alternatively, we should acknowledge that the five outcomes do facilitate personal development and may therefore provide the opportunity for spiritual growth.

ACTIVITY

Consider the five outcomes listed in *Every Child Matters* (2004):

1. being healthy
2. staying safe
3. enjoying and achieving
4. making a positive contribution
5. economic wellbeing

Do you think that the children in your care are enabled to achieve spiritual fulfilment with the above agenda?

Could it be that many adults who provide care for children are unaware or afraid of the notion of spirituality, and focus their attention on physical management only? Many care providers in the health care arena consider that the spiritual needs of the child should be addressed by the 'local vicar' and they are not the responsibility of nurses and care workers. Pfund (2000) argues that health care professionals need to have the listening skills to hear what the child has to say, and the courage and imagination to respond. It would be wrong to expect a religious leader of any faith to be entirely responsible for the child/family's ability to express such needs. Surely we should be reminded of our holistic focus of care by such seminal texts as that by Roper *et al.* (1980), which directs health care workers to provide individualized holistic care, albeit within a reductionist framework. Families and children who express no faith will also need to be facilitated to express their inner spirituality, and this may not 'fit' with any spiritual leader's role. It could also be argued that,with such involvement, the health professional may grow personally by joining in the child and family's journey through their spiritual expression and need, thus enriching their own professional role.

Challenges of children's palliative care

For many children who receive palliative care within the hospice environment, spirituality may be a key focus of care. Certain aspects of the ethos of this environment mean there is 'time to be' and there may be 'freedom of expression'. These may be high priority, but even then the care staff may feel poorly prepared for the challenges that spiritual communication may present. One reflective question practitioners and carers may want to ask is: do we really want to hear what the child has to say? The opportunity to be involved in care for children and families at the end of the children's lives is a challenge and a privilege, but we cannot expect to be unchanged by such involvement. Therefore health care professionals and carers may be faced with some challenges with regard to spiritual care. An important question to explore and address within all children's palliative care services is: How may health professionals facilitate expression of self and spirituality?

Could it be that the child who becomes very relaxed and has a smile on his or her face while in a warm Jacuzzi is not only enjoying the warmth but also expressing inner peace and freedom from anxiety and pain. Is this spiritual care? Imaginative play with paints and water may enable a child to produce something that is a visualization of his or her inner thoughts; music and sensory room time may also provide relaxation but also time to be, to think and to feel.

Storytelling is a well recognized format for providing information for children and to allow situations to be explained and reinforced (discussed in Chapter 3). The use of the same text that the child enjoys can provide a sense of security and inner peace. Witte-Townsend and DiGiulio (2004: 127) suggest that 'the reading and rereading of familiar stories enables understanding of complex human issues and contributes significantly to social, emotional and spiritual growth'. Storytelling is usually a familiar communication method for children and families, and can also assist in giving information – this may be a useful method of spiritual communication between carer and child.

Music therapy or simply making a noise may also provide many children with the means to express inner fears as well as happiness. Such activities as loud noise or soothing melody would be familiar within any paediatric environment and are especially important not only for the child who is ill but also for his or her carers and siblings. Such activities provide an opportunity to let out inner feelings or to feel at peace with the world.

Many hospice communities regularly use the skills of the Pets As Therapy dogs (PAT 2008). This enables children to touch, see, feel and smell another living creature, which can provide a much needed opportunity to feel free and influence the movement and mood of a responsive being. For many children, their condition or disease process means that they spend most of the day having actions 'done to them', such as caring interventions and procedures. The PAT dogs and other pet therapy can help to counterbalance this. A child who has felt the pleasure of a dog laying its head on his or her lap while being stroked can feel much reward and self-satisfaction. Is this a form of spiritual care?

Limitations to providing spiritual care

Palliative care for children also presents a further challenge to the carer in relation to age and development. Developmental stage is often more crucial than the age of the child when considering communication and understanding of the world and all it contains for the child. Consideration must also be given to the restrictions that are faced by those giving palliative care within an acute care environment. Children may be admitted to the acute ward where the parents, staff and child know each other well. This may provide the sense of security and individuality that the child and family require, but the busy nature of the ward may prevent the time being available to deliver 'spiritual care'. Indeed, the time required by the family may place added strain on the acute care staff, who find they are not able to give their full attention to the needs of the child and feel a sense of frustration as a result. Accordingly, many acute care environments have developed links with palliative care teams to provide some additional support, either in the acute environment or by transferring the child to the palliative care facility.

KEY POINT

Developmental stage is often more crucial than the age of the child when considering communication and understanding of the world and all it contains for the child.

Conclusion

Spirituality is a fundamental aspect of children's palliative care services. Children may experience and express their spiritual needs in different ways depending on their age and stage of development. Much of the research undertaken into explaining and exploring spirituality and spiritual care has been derived from adult perspectives, with adult services in mind. The challenge for all who are working within children's or paediatric palliative care services is to transfer the rhetoric, developments and recommendations surrounding spirituality, spiritual need and spiritual care from adult-orientated services into their own clinical context so that this will have meaning and significance for the children and families for whom they care.

Key resources

Kenny, G. (1999) The iron cage and the spider's web: children's spirituality and the hospital environment. *Paediatric Nursing* **11**(5): 20–3.

McSherry, W. (2006) *Making Sense of Spirituality in Nursing and Health Care Practice: An Interactive Approach,* 2nd edn. London: Jessica Kingsley.

Pfund, R. (2000) Nurturing a child's spirituality. *Journal of Child Health Nursing* **4**(4): 143–8.

CHAPTER SUMMARY

■ The concept of spirituality is firmly embedded within health care practice.

■ There is no agreed definition of what constitutes spirituality; it is complex, multi-faceted and can be viewed in different ways.

■ In comparison to adults, spirituality is expressed and experienced more at an emotional level.

■ There is a need for inter-/intra-disciplinary working; no health care profession has a monopoly with regards to this aspect of care. Collaboration and interprofessional dialogue are required so that children's palliative care services acknowledge the importance of this dimension of care.

■ Practitioners and carers working within children's palliative care need to engage with the general language and debates surrounding spirituality and spiritual care. This will foster their understanding of this within their own specialist areas.

■ Spiritual and religious care must be sensitive and respectful of the child and the family. It must not be imposing and intrusive; it should be integrated within the 'general' services and day- to- day care delivery.

■ Spiritual care is not an addition or about doing, it is about presence and being with children and families as they struggle with and try to make sense of the situations they experience.

References

Anandarajah, G. and Hight, E. (2001) spirituality and medical practice: using the HOPE questions as a practical tool for spiritual assessment. *American Family Physician* **63**(1): 81–8.

Anderson, B. and Steen, S. (1995) Spiritual care reflecting God's love to children. *Journal of Christian Nursing* **12**(2): 12–17, 47.

Dawkins, R. (2006) *The GOD Delusion.* London: Bantam.

DH (Department of Health) (2003) NHS *Chaplaincy: Meeting the Religious and Spiritual Needs of Patients and Staff.* London: Department of Health.

DH (Department of Health) (2004) *National Service Framework for Children, Every Child Matters.* London: Department of Health.

Doka, K. J. (1994) Suffer the little children: the child and spirituality in the AIDS crisis. In Pfund, R. (2000) Nurturing a child's spirituality. *Journal of Child Health Care* **4**(4): 143–8.

Erikson, E. H. (1963) *Childhood and Society*, 2nd edn. New York: W. W. Norton.

Gilliat-Ray, S. (2001) Sociological perspectives on the pastoral care of minority faiths in hospital. In Orchard, H. (ed.) *Spirituality in Health Care Contexts.* London: Jessica Kingsley, pp. 135–46.

Henley, A. and Schott, J. (1999) *Culture, Religion and Patient Care in a Multi-Ethnic Society.* London: Age Concern.

Hull, J. (1998) Religious education and the spiritual rights of children. In Watson, J. (2006) *Every Child Matters* and children's spiritual rights: does the new holistic approach to children's care address children's spiritual well being? *International Journal of Children's Spirituality* **11**(2): 251–63.

Kenny, G. and Ashley, M. (2005) Children's student nurses' knowledge of spirituality and its implications for educational practice. *Journal of Child Health Care* **9**(3): 174–85.

Kenny, G. (1999) The iron cage and the spider's web: children's spirituality and the hospital environment. *Paediatric Nursing* **11**(5): 20–3.

Koenig, H. G., McCullough, M. E. and Larson, D. B. (2001) *Handbook of Religion and Health*. Oxford: Oxford University Press.

McSherry, W. and Ross, L. (2002) Dilemmas of spiritual assessment: considerations for nursing practice. *Journal of Advanced Nursing* **38**(5): 479–88.

McSherry, W. and Smith, J. (2007) How do children express their spiritual needs? *Paediatric Nursing* **19**(3): 17–20.

McSherry, W. (2006) *Making Sense of Spirituality in Nursing and Health Care Practice: An Interactive Approach*, 2nd edn. London: Jessica Kingsley.

Murray, R. B. and Zentner, J. B. (1989) *Nursing concepts for health promotion*. London: Prentice Hall.

Narayanasamy, A. (2001) *Spiritual Care: A Practical Guide for Nurses and Health Care Practitioners*, 2nd edn. London: Quay Books.

Neuberger, J. (2004) *Caring for Dying People of Different Faiths*, 3rd edn. Oxford: Radcliffe Publishing.

NICE (National Institute for Health and Clinical Excellence) (2004) *Improving Supportive and Palliative Care for Adults with Cancer*. London: NICE.

Nursing and Midwifery Council (2004) *Requirements for Pre-Registration Nursing Programmes*. London: NMC.

Pets As Therapy (2008) Available at: www.petsastherapy.org; accessed 29 February 2008.

Pfund, R. (2000) Nurturing a child's spirituality. *Journal of Child Health Nursing* **4**(4): 143–8.

Piaget, J. (1952) *The Origins of Intelligence in Children*. New York: International Universities Press.

Puchalski, C. and Romer, A. L. (2002) Taking a spiritual history allows clinicians to understand patients more fully. *Journal of Palliative Medicine* **3**(1): 129–37.

Roper, N., Logan, W., and Tierney, A. (1980) *The Roper Logan and Tierney Model of Nursing: Based on Activities of Daily Living*. Oxford: Churchill Livingstone.

Schneider, M. A. and Mannell, R. C. (2006) Beacon in the storm: an exploration of the spirituality and faith of parents whose children have cancer. *Issues in Comprehensive Pediatric Nursing* **29**: 3–24.

Scottish Executive Health Department (2002) *Guidelines on Chaplaincy and Spiritual Care in the NHS Scotland* (NHS HDL (2002) 76). Edinburgh: Scottish Executive.

Seden, J. (1998) The spiritual needs of children. *Practice* **10**(4): 57–67.

Smith, J. and McSherry, W. (2004) Spirituality and child development: a concept analysis. *Journal of Advanced Nursing* **45**(3): 307–15.

Steen, S. and Anderson, B. (1995) Ages and stages of spiritual development. *Journal of Christian Nursing* **12**(2): 6–11.

Turner, P. (1996) Caring more, doing less. *Nursing Times* **92**(34): 59–60.

Watson, J. (2006) *Every Child Matters* and children's spiritual rights: does the new holistic approach to children's care address children's spiritual well being? *International Journal of Children's Spirituality* **11**(2): 251–63.

Witte-Townsend, D. L. and DiGiulio, E. (2004) Something for nothing: exploring dimensions of children's knowing through the repeated reading of favourite books. *International Journal of Children's Spirituality* **9**(2): 127–42.

WHO (World Health Organization) (2008) *WHO Definition of Palliative Care for Children*. Available at: www.who.int/cancer/palliative/definition/en/print.html; accessed 18 April 2008.

6

Supporting Children and Families

Fiona Collinson and Karen Bleakley

Introduction

As discussed in the first chapter of this book, the numbers of life-limited and life-threatened children are increasing on a global scale. Children are living with more complex conditions requiring skilled, time-consuming and stressful interventions (Mencap 2001, SCN 2003), often carried out in their own home (Kirk and Glendinning 2002). This undoubtedly places further demands on parents, families and existing support services. Evidence regarding the detrimental physical, social, emotional and financial effects on carers and siblings is widely reported (O'Brien 2001, Valkinier *et al.* 2002, DfES and DH 2004) and the relentlessness of having this responsibility is documented in many studies (Hartnick *et al.* 2003, Redmond and Richardson 2003, Montagnino and Mauricio 2004). Previous studies have highlighted the importance of support provided by the health care team, and parents often recount the support they received from specific individuals (Brody and Simmons 2007). However, the provision of support is a challenging issue for service providers. Such challenges range from individual and family perspectives of recognizing the need for support, to organizational issues of recruitment, training and retention of appropriate staff.

Recognition of the need for support is documented at statutory, voluntary and government levels within the UK. Most recently, the 'Every disabled child matters' agenda has highlighted the need for ongoing support as a mechanism to help each child reach his or her potential (HM Treasury and DfES 2007). While there is no doubt that caring for disabled children is particularly challenging, it should be acknowledged that, despite many difficulties, some studies have revealed the positive or rewarding aspects of caring for these families (see, for example, Redmond and Richardson 2003).

While families' requirements and the availability of services vary across hospital, hospice and home settings, this topic is discussed in Chapter 9 and therefore will not be repeated here. It is also acknowledged that, in order to meet the needs of children and families, health care professionals themselves need support via a range of mechanisms, as highlighted in Chapter 10. The aim of this chapter is to explore the types of support that children and parents may require. First, however, it is necessary to consider the nature of support and when it may be required.

Psychosocial support

Psychosocial support is an umbrella term for a range of support mechanisms. Numerous definitions of support are discussed by Cook (1999), but essentially it is assistance in a practical, emotional or financial manner which alleviates the physical, social and emotional stresses experienced by an individual child and/or family. These stresses result from the physical, social and psychological impact of the child's illness, its cause, duration and progression. Stress is a demand on an individual's physical or mental energy and is a problem when it becomes overwhelming. We all employ different coping strategies to enable us to deal with life events, and this in itself can cause family conflict if parents deal with their child's illness in differing ways. Stress and the types of coping strategies are very specific to families and individuals (Cook 1999), though it is recognized that more resilient families cope better with crises and overcome the challenges they face (Brody and Simmons 2007). In a recent study by Beresford, Rabiee and Sloper (2007; see Further Reading box below), parents indicated that they wanted support to enable them to be a parent to their child and not just a carer or nurse, to reduce the emotional impact of the situation for themselves, to enable them to do things as a family, and to preserve the mother–father relationship.

══════ FURTHER READING ══════

Read Beresford, B., Rabiee, P. and Sloper, P. (2007) *Priorities and Perceptions of Disabled Children and Young People and Their Parents Regarding Outcomes from Support Services.* York: Social Policy Research Unit. Available at: www.york.ac.ujk/inst/spru/research/pdf/priorities.pdf

Consider how the findings of this study inform the further development of support services in your area.

When is psychosocial support needed?

Psychosocial support begins at the time of diagnosis (which could be prenatal) or from initial symptom appearance, and should continue throughout the illness, end-of-life care, death and bereavement. The impending death of a child within a family shakes that group to its core, affecting all those associated. The composition of families today is ever-changing. Often families may be reconstituted as a result of relationships failing and include parents, partners, step-parents, stepchildren and half siblings, and frequently several generations of a family are involved. Steele (2005) found that families 'put life on hold' when their child became ill, had difficulty in maintaining friendships outside the family and, with everything focused around the child's needs, family life became very regimented. Therefore, the type and amount of psychosocial support required is unique to each individual and family. Professionals need to recognize that each individual determines his/her own 'family', acknowledging that connections may be genetic, legal or emotional. Parental responsibility for the child should always be clarified, as individual circumstances will dictate to whom and from whom information should be given and sought.

═══════════════════════ **ACTIVITY** ═══════════════════════

Reflect on a family you have worked with. Who constituted the family for the child, parent and yourself?

The need for support is influenced by many factors (see Figure 6.1). Everyone has pre-existing coping mechanisms that have developed as a result of their life experiences. A great deal has been written about recognized gender differences such as females being more emotive and males more practical, but as Martin and Doka (2000) highlight, these responses are not always gender-specific. The interdisciplinary team should recognize this and be aware that previous experiences of illness, disability and death have a great impact on individuals' coping skills. A major area affecting family support requirements is the particular illness or disability the child may have, and the resulting physical care, prognosis and time span involved in the care of the child (DfES and DH 2004, Standard 5). Social support

---

▩   Pre-existing coping mechanisms

▩   Previous experiences

▩   Gender

▩   Child's illness/disability

▩   Social support networks

▩   Culture

▩   Environment

▩   Socio-economic background

▩   Age and developmental stage of children in family

▩   Parenting capacity

▩   Level of understanding of situation and ability

Figure 6.1   Some of the factors influencing the need for support

networks vary greatly between families and may be influenced by ethnic and cultural background and beliefs. Environmental factors such as appropriate housing, transport and geographical location are significant components affecting the provision of support.

It is important to recognize that families do not always accept help initially: therefore, as a minimum standard, they should be provided with a written record of relevant contact numbers, including 'out of hours' services, enabling the family to access services when they are ready. The variation in need, type and amount of support for families is unquantifiable, and may mean different things to different professionals and families, oscillating throughout the duration of the illness, and depending on its length (NICE 2005). Some families need practical care and support twenty-four hours a day, while others merely need to know that advice is available.

━━━━━━━━━━━━━━ **FURTHER READING** ━━━━━━━━━━━━━━

Read Brett, J. (2004) The journey to accepting support: how parents of profoundly disabled children experience support in their lives. *Paediatric Nursing* **16**(8): 14–18.

Consider the support experienced by these parents and compare this to the parents you encounter in your own practice.

Assessment

An accurate and comprehensive assessment is essential to ensure that the needs of a life-limited/life-threatened child and family are the focus for the interdisciplinary team. The child's key worker is ideally placed to co-ordinate the completion of this, with involvement from other relevant professionals who acquire information for the assessment from the family, share this with interdisciplinary colleagues and thereby contribute to a holistic assessment. This eclectic and family-centred approach to assessment should ensure that services are 'needs led' and avoid duplication, or repetition, for parents. It should also indicate the type of support required by each family, and clarify the degree of involvement families want to have in care and decision-making.

An assessment should address the strengths and weaknesses/problems of a child and family's situation and how these influence their coping abilities. Physical, environmental, behavioural, emotional, financial and social factors and their implications for treatment and care are included, with cultural, spiritual and faith beliefs being inherent throughout the process (see Figure 6.2).

Despite its comprehensive nature, the framework in Figure 6.2 does not address specifically the complex needs of children with life-limiting conditions. Initially, the family may not know what they need or what is available. In response to this, ACT have produced further assessment guidelines (ACT, 2003) which aim to build up and establish a holistic picture of the complex needs of children with disabilities and/or life-limiting conditions and those of their families. Professionals have a responsibility to inform and advise families of possible support services, and ensure that the process is supportive and not invasive. Individual assessments

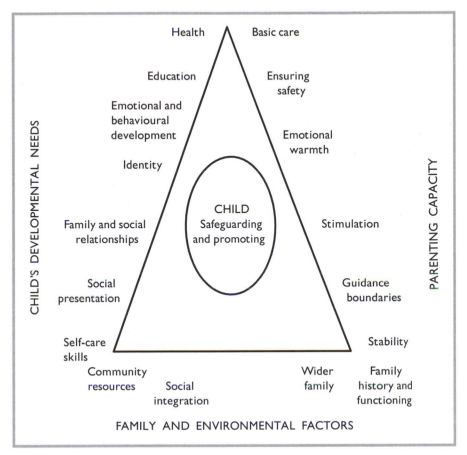

Figure 6.2 Framework for assessment of children in need and their families

Source: Department for Children, Schools and Families (2000, p. 17).

Crown copyright is reproduced with the permission of the Controller of HMSO and Queen's Printer for Scotland.

must be performed when a family is referred to support services initially and on a regular planned basis thereafter (NICE 2005). The provision and receipt of support should be seen as a responsive, ever-changing process. This includes the time after the initial contact, at times of change, on discharge from hospital, when curative treatment is no longer feasible, or if the family or professional identify a change in the perceived need for support. Care pathways such as the ACT care pathway (ACT 2004) provide a structure to facilitate the organization of support mechanisms.

FURTHER READING

Read ACT (Association for Children with Life-Threatening or Terminal Conditions and their Families) (2003) *Assessment of Children with Life Limiting Conditions and Their Families. A Guide to Effective Care Planning*. Bristol: ACT; and ACT (Association for Children with Life-threatening or Terminal Conditions and their Families) (2004) *Integrated Multi-Agency Care Pathways for Children with Life-Threatening and Life-Limiting Conditions*. Bristol: ACT;

both available at: www.act.org.uk) and consider if your current practice reflects the guidance recommended in these documents.

Types of support

Support is highlighted as one of the most important factors that help children's carers to cope during difficult periods (McGrath 2001). Many parents of life-limited/life-threatened children find it difficult to acknowledge their need for support and resist doing so, often viewing this as a sign of failure on their part (Brett 2004). Formal support from health care professionals is recognized as important, but more informal support provided by family, friends and other parents is also viewed as being significant to parents (McGrath 2001). Support can be divided broadly into three interconnected components – emotional, practical and financial – with the provision of information being central to them all (Kirk and Glendinning 2002, Beresford, Adshead and Croft, 2007, Kerr *et al.* 2007). The information needs of the child and family are discussed in Chapter 3 and are therefore not explored further here.

There are many different associations, both nationally and locally, that may be approached for support. Organizations may be illness specific – for example, CLIC Sargent and Macmillan Cancer Support, which care for children with cancer, The Society for Mucopolysaccharide Diseases, the Cystic Fibrosis Trust, the Muscular Dystrophy Campaign – or more general – for example, the Family Fund. Contact a Family produce an invaluable directory of information regarding specific conditions and rare disorders, and provide links to the relevant organizations. Websites also provide an overview of services, but local knowledge of available resources should not be overlooked. The regional variations in these are often a source of frustration to families, but these can be alleviated by a knowledgeable and resourceful guide from within the interdisciplinary team.

KEY POINT

Support can be divided broadly into three interconnected components emotional, practical and financial with the provision of information being central to them all.

Emotional support

Families receiving paediatric palliative care are 'normal' families in 'abnormal' situations as a result of the illness of their child (Edwards and Davis 1997). It is important that they have someone to approach who can provide advice and support, or to direct them to an appropriate professional. Research shows that children and families rated being able to talk openly about their feelings as being of extreme importance (Jones 2006) and that 'the reassurance that someone out there cares' (McGrath 2001: 201) also provided much support. Many children and families benefit from receiving emotional support, enabling them to discuss their feelings in confidence, but it should also be recognized that not everyone finds such support useful (McGrath 2001). Families will talk when the time is 'right' for them. Indeed, studies have identified that it is beneficial for families to have a professional with whom they can express their feelings, can trust to listen, is non-judgmental, and who they know will maintain their confidentiality (Kirk and Glendinning 2002, Beresford, Rabiee and Sloper 2007).

Emotional support is often sought through counselling, which can be provided by professional, specifically-trained counsellors, and by others who use counselling skills in their wider roles for example, teachers, nurses and social workers. Studies have indicated that non-professional counsellors can be as effective as professional ones (McLeod 2000) and it is the qualities of the person providing this type of support that makes it effective. Opportunities for families to talk to other families with similar issues can be 'better than professional counselling' (McGrath 2001: 202) and mutually beneficial (Redmond and Richardson,2003). This can be formal, in the form of parent support groups or informal; for example, meeting other parents during mealtimes (Redmond and Richardson 2003).

WEB LINKS

Search the resource: www.cafamily.org.uk and find out what advice is available for families caring for a child who requires palliative care.

Many theoretical models of counselling exist, but when using a family-centred approach to paediatric palliative care, Carl Rogers' work should be considered. Rogers (1951) developed the 'person-centred' approach to counselling, identifying three core conditions – empathy, congruence and acceptance – that need to exist within a therapeutic relationship for it to be beneficial. He believed that the therapeutic relationship between client and counsellor was paramount, that the client is the expert and the counsellor's role is to facilitate change within the client through use of active empathic listening, reflection and unconditional positive regard. This therapeutic relationship is based on trust, good interpersonal skills, an understanding of the family's situation and the wider implications for them. The counsellor's personal beliefs and attitudes, character and personality are all of importance (McLeod 2000). Working within paediatric palliative care, most members of the interdisciplinary team will use a variety of counselling skills within their daily practice, albeit at different levels depending on their training, role and experience. They should be able to identify normal reactions in stressful situations and have a knowledge of loss and bereavement theories and the grieving process. It is essential staff that are able to recognize if a family's experiences are outside of the 'normal' range, when more expert support, in the form of onward referral to specialist mental health services, is required (Edwards and Davis 1997).

The support provided by hospital staff in terms of provision of information, emotional support and practical care is invaluable (McGrath 2001), though hospitals are often associated with negative events – for example, diagnosis, crises/episodes of ill-health – and wards have been described as a 'goldfish bowl where everyone knows everything' (Hewitt-Taylor 2008: 110). Home visits are extremely important, with families and children often more willing to talk as they are in a familiar environment which is their 'own space'. Confidentiality should be maintained throughout the professional–family relationship; however, it is each professional's responsibility to be aware of situations when client confidentiality may need to be breached – for example child protection issues.

Financial support

Recent estimates indicate that over 90 per cent of disabled children live at home with their families, with 55 per cent of these families surviving in or on the margins of poverty. Furthermore, it is thought that it costs three times more to raise a disabled child than a non-disabled one (Dobson *et al.* 2001). Household income is inevitably affected, as few families have budgeted for the expenses involved in having a sick child, either at home or in hospital, and for providing constant care for whatever length of time. In most families, one or both parents may be unable to work because of the complex care needs of their child (Carers UK 2007) but yet 'life goes on' and bills have to be paid regardless of other issues. Routine payments on mortgages, rent, loans and so on have to be maintained while meeting additional costs of travelling to and from hospital, car parking, maintaining a family home and living in hospital, increased home heating, and maintaining and powering equipment.

The social worker within the interdisciplinary team usually undertakes a detailed financial assessment with the family to provide a record of their income and expenditure, and identify areas of financial concern and strain. It is important to check out financial circumstances in a sensitive and discreet manner, as families are often reluctant to divulge this information. Financial assistance may be available from statutory and voluntary organizations, but families must be made aware that an assessment of financial means is often a prerequisite when making these applications, and the information provided must be accurate. Applications tend to be means-tested and though not necessarily dependent on a family receiving qualifying state benefits, all have their individual criteria. If specific equipment is required, it is always worthwhile applying on behalf of a family as any award received will be beneficial. Support available may include annual grants towards items for the child, family holidays, home heating costs, home insulation schemes, clothing, activities or play/education equipment.

Employers should be kept informed; mortgage lenders may offer 'mortgage holidays' in some circumstances, and critical illness insurance cover may include children, but all these need to be checked out individually. Social workers will advocate on behalf of children and families, liaising with benefits agencies, completing forms and providing letters of support. Local Citizens Advice Bureaux and Welfare Rights offices provide guidance with benefits agencies, providing helpline numbers and advice on specific benefits.

Disability Living Allowance (DLA)

DLA is a non-means-tested state benefit for which life-limited/ life-threatened children may be eligible. This benefit is not awarded on diagnosis, but on the amount of physical care, support and supervision a child with an illness or disability needs compared to a child of a similar age without such an illness/disability. Children aged three and over may also receive the mobility component of DLA if appropriate. Families on benefits may be eligible for extra allowances if their child receives DLA. Amount awarded, the duration of the award and the reviewing of this varies, and professionals should be aware that this is frequently a source of great distress to families, who often have to wait an undue length of time for money when their income is restricted or expenditure increased.

Direct payments

Direct payments must be offered to parents of disabled children to allow them greater flexibility and choice as to how they receive support services (OPSI 2001). However, there is no national framework to standardize eligibility criteria for these, and each local authority/health care trust sets its own criteria and is responsible for the prioritizing of provision of payments. Payment is based on the individual assessment of circumstances by community-based social services. Some families choose to receive payments directly and use this money to arrange their own care. Any carer has the right to request an assessment of their own needs (DH 2000), which then enables them to avail themselves of this service. In principle, direct payments should provide families with the means of acquiring a flexible service that is responsive to their needs.

WEB LINKS

Search these resources and find out what advice is available for families caring for a child who requires palliative care: Citizens Advice Bureau – available at: www.citizensadvice.org; Department for Work and Pensions – available at: www.dwp.gov.uk; and Assessment for carers and Direct payments – available at: www.direct.gov.uk

Practical support

Practical support takes many forms – from a neighbour or relative collecting siblings from school, to general housework. While such practical help is not always needed, the fact that it is available is a comfort to many parents (Brody and Simmons 2007). Professionals from both the statutory and voluntary sectors should enable families to recognize the type of support they require, and give the families choices and options.

ACTIVITY

List some ways that a non-trained family member could support a family in a practical manner.

Often, a child requires such a vast range of equipment and specialized care that there is a risk that parents may lose their parenting role to that of being an unqualified but highly trained carer (Aldridge 2007). The provision of specialized equipment requires appropriate and timely referral to relevant community-based professionals – for example, occupational therapist (OT), physiotherapist, community nurse (MENCAP 2001) – who will provide a professional report in support of any request for financial assistance. A vast range of equipment is required for life-limited/life-threatened children, which needs to be ordered. Specialized equipment is not a luxury; it is a necessity to enable children and families to achieve as high a quality of life as possible. Delays in ordering and receiving customized equipment, such as wheelchairs, may mean that the item is no longer suitable by the time it arrives. Families, lay carers and the interdisciplinary team caring for the child need specific training in using and maintaining relevant equipment, as well as mandatory training such as moving and handling. Many families will require home adaptations, or even have to relocate. A thorough assessment of a family's situation and knowledge of the child's potential future needs will determine the adaptations required. These should be anticipated early, to ensure that the home is suitable for the child and carers when the physical needs arise. Housing adaptations for children with long-term needs are not means tested, but there is a financial limit. An effective working partnership between the family, occupational therapist and housing department is necessary, as is illustrated in the clinical focus example below.

CLINICAL FOCUS

Luke is a 10-year-old boy with muscular dystrophy, who attends a mainstream school. He has been known to the occupational therapy department since diagnosis at the age of 7, and seen regularly for review appointments. Luke lives with his mother and two sisters in a semi-detached house. Luke's mobility has recently deteriorated and he has now become dependent on his wheelchair. It is very difficult for Luke to manoeuvre around the house in his wheelchair as there are steps at both the front and back doors, the house has narrow doorways, and Luke's bedroom and the bathroom are located upstairs. The family made a temporary ramp for the steps to the back door. Some time ago the idea of altering the home environment to meet Luke's changing needs was introduced. This was not a welcomed or well-received suggestion. Luke's mother did not wish to consider permanent adaptations to her home, as she was finding it difficult to acknowledge the deterioration in Luke's condition, and accepting the necessity of the change would further highlight this deterioration. Only bathing aids were accepted to aid in Luke's day-to-day care.
He continued to grow and he became increasingly dependent on his mother, who attended to all his daily needs. She has now approached the OT Department requesting assistance with housing adaptations.

INTERDISCIPLINARY INSIGHT

Role of the occupational therapist in Luke's care

- Regular review of child at home/clinic/school.

- Timely assessment and provision of equipment, including specialized buggies/manual or powered wheelchairs, specialized seating, toileting aids, bathing aids and so on, as negotiated with the child and family.

- Advice to family and respite providers regarding manual handling, equipment issues.

- Assessment of child's needs around housing adaptations, in partnership with child and his parents/carers and liaising with the housing department.

- Timely initiation of recommendations for disabled facilities grant.

- Provision of information and signposting to other resources and services as required.

- Close liaison with interdisciplinary team.

- Assessment of school environment with recommendations for specialized equipment/ adaptations as required.

- Contribution to statement of educational needs.

- Ongoing support of child and family.

Written by Jill Clarke, Children's Occupational Therapist.

Accessible and appropriate transport is a also a necessity to prevent families becoming isolated; specialized car seating may progress to the need for adapted transport; both of which add to the cost of caring for a child, but assist families to maintain their independence. The mobility component of DLA is awarded in recognition of the extra costs associated with transportation. It can be offset against the cost of a vehicle or towards suitable public transport, and allows the family to apply for a disabled parking badge and road tax exemption. Hospital staff should advise families on parking facilities, car parking fees and concessions available.

=== **ACTIVITY** ===

Consider a technology-dependent, life-limited/life-threatened child you have cared for. List the equipment used and the training required to care for this child in the community.

Respite

A major component in the area of practical support is the provision of respite care, the aims of which are set out in Figure 6.3. Respite is getting rest or relief; in fact a 'true break' from the care routine and associated stresses. Laverty and Reet (2001) recommend that families should be empowered through respite, and siblings shielded from being overwhelmed by the shadow of the child with complex needs. Respite care is a vital service, a necessity rather than a luxury (NICHCY 2005) and families should have access to a range of flexible and individualized respite care (RCN 2005, Corkin *et al.* 2006) on a regular basis.

The terminology used can often have negative implications for families (Murphy 2001, Thurgate 2004), particularly the term respite (Weightman 2000). Professionals have a responsibility to ensure that alternative terms used to describe respite care, such as 'short break', are acceptable and positive to the individual families, and that families understand the service offered.

The aims of respite care

■ To support the family in the care of their child in the community.

■ To enable the child or young person to have a break from their family with appropriate support, to have fun and to interact at a level appropriate for them.

■ To allow families to have a break from the caring routine, and enable them to maintain a social support network.

■ To provide opportunities for siblings to have fun and receive support in their own right.

Respite care may offer the whole family an opportunity to be together and to be supported in the care of their child, or it may offer care solely for the child or young person.

Figure 6.3 The aims of respite care

=========================== ACTIVITY ===========================

Consider the term respite; does it have positive or negative connotations for you?

The availability of appropriate respite care

Many studies of families caring for technologically dependant children, or those who have disabilities, have reported their need for respite (Damiani *et al.* 2004). The provision of appropriate respite care must be available to families before they reach 'breaking point'; however, there are many inconsistencies in service provision and inequities of service throughout the United Kingdom. Appropriate statutory respite care for children requiring palliative care is scarce, as traditional respite services were designed for children with developmental or behavioural problems rather than those with complex nursing needs (While *et al.* 1996). Thankfully, this situation is changing with the recent announcement of a multi-million pound investment in England for short-break services by the Department for Children, Schools and Families and the Aiming High for Disabled Children programme (HM Treasury and DfES 2007). Managers and practitioners working in this area are aware that it is often families most in need, children with significant nursing and medical requirements for whom it is the most difficult to provide support, and who wait the longest for the service (Mencap 2003) (SCN 2003). Support provision for evenings, nights, weekends and school holidays is difficult, as staff are often reluctant to work anti-social hours.

Benefits and limitations of respite care

Respite care provision gives families the opportunity to do the ordinary things that others take for granted. Families who receive good respite services perceive them as a 'lifeline' (Bleakley 2008) and while parental stress cannot be fully removed, respite care can reduce it (Cowen and Reed 2002). Respite care services should provide planned support as well as catering for emergency situations (Olsen and Maslin-Prothero 2001, Bleakley 2008). Parents value having trained and experienced nurses and carers providing respite care in their own homes, but needed consistency and continuity of care to develop trust in the professionals involved (Bleakley 2008). Respite care that in reality or in parents' perception does not match the care they provide may increase their stress (Robinson *et al.* 2001). Some parents may have feelings of guilt (Nicoll *et al.* 2002, Hartrey and Wells 2003) or safety concerns when using respite. Being time-conscious spoils the enjoyment of having a break for some parents (Steele 2005) or, as Nicoll *et al.* (2002: 479) point out, 'the carer may feel marooned and directionless without the imperative of daily caring duties', which highlights the importance of families receiving respite care before losing their social support network.

The provision of respite care

Those managing respite care provision have a great responsibility to recruit, train, retain and support staff in whom parents will have confidence. Key issues in respite care provision are included in Figure 6.4. Attracting the 'right' person who is, or who can be, trained to a level of competence, be knowledgeable and skilled to look after these precious children regularly and for a potentially long time is challenging. It is difficult to attract and retain registered nurses in this area, and expensive and time-consuming to train care assistants. Staff are also required to have a personality that is acceptable to the child and the parents, and in the case of staff in the community, to be able to work alone, make decisions regarding care, and be flexible to the individual situations they might find themselves in. The lack of access to skilled, competent staff is a significant issue apparent to managers, as reported by Parker *et al.* (1999). Often as a result of training issues, respite care may have to be timed around the child using equipment (Heaton *et al.* 2005) or requiring medication (Bleakley 2008). In a study by Neufeld *et al.* (2001), one mother recounted that most of her respite allocation was spent training staff, who then might not have been available when the family needed respite.

The need for paediatric palliative care in any family will have repercussions for all those close to the child. Family life is disrupted whether following the birth of a life-limited child or the diagnosis of a life-threatening illness. Extended family, friends and the local community will share this unique and distressing situation. In particular, the needs of siblings and grandparents are often overlooked.

Sibling support

Siblings of children with palliative care needs have often grown up in the shadow of illness as their parents, as a matter of priority, focus on the needs of their sick child. Siblings' needs (including those of full, half or stepsiblings) are understandably viewed as being less important, often at an emotional and psychological cost to them – a 'benign neglect' (Edwards and Davis 1997: 183). Their routines and

- Continuity – staff must be known to the both the child and parents.

- Parents need to trust staff.

- Parents must be confident that staff are knowledgeable regarding their child – personality, condition, potential emergency situations.

- Available back-up staff known to family.

- Type of respite – choice for family.

- Duration of the 'break' must be sufficient.

- Easy to organise (from the parent's perspective).

- Frequency – regular/when family need it.

- Flexible (planned and emergency).

- Available weekends, evenings and during school holidays.

- Free.

- Local.

- Effective communication between the child, family and services.

- Enjoyable experience.

- Family respite unit to enable the family to stay together if they so wish.

- Early intervention to prevent long-term effect on family social networks.

Figure 6.4   Key issues in the provision of respite care

home life may be badly affected, and parents may not be available to them – physically or emotionally. Some siblings feel different from their peers (Brown 2007) and may feel frightened, guilty, anxious and unsure as to what is expected of them. However, this is not always the case, and many children cope well if they are informed, involved and supported, particularly at difficult times when their parents' attentions may be diverted elsewhere. Siblings' coping mechanisms are affected by their age and stage of development, their understanding of the situation and their past experiences, but mainly from learnt behaviour from within the family. Parents are usually best placed to talk to siblings about what is happening, and members of the interdisciplinary team should enable them to do so, and provide them with information, support and guidance. Advice for parents is included in Figure 6.5.

Siblings should be involved directly in the assessment process, to gain an insight into their specific needs. A practical and fun way of doing this is to use an Ecomap (Parker and Bradley, 2007). This gives structure to the assessment and an immediate picture of the children and their relationships/sources of support within the family. Children draw a circle in the middle with their name in it and add other circles to represent others in their life. Lines are drawn between circles indicating

Sibling support – suggestions for parents

- Be open and honest from outset with siblings preparing them for times ahead.

- Make time for siblings

- Build upon their past experiences of illness and loss wherever possible.

- It is acceptable not to know the answer – some questions don't have answers – what is important is that siblings have the opportunity to ask.

- Establish and maintain a routine for siblings, providing them with a sense of security, e.g. a parent is at home at bedtime whenever possible. Record this on a calendar.

- Reassure siblings that it is OK for them to have fun, be with friends, etc.

- Ensure siblings have regular contact with each other, this could be through phone calls, texts, e-mails, etc. if direct contact is not possible

- Keep school informed – school often provides a stable and constant environment for children outside of their 'abnormal' family situation. Schools now have staff dedicated to pastoral care of students and have access to school counsellors.

- Liaise with relevant members of interdisciplinary team for guidance on available resources to facilitate 'difficult' conversations (see McNeilly and Price, 2008)

Figure 6.5   Advice for parents

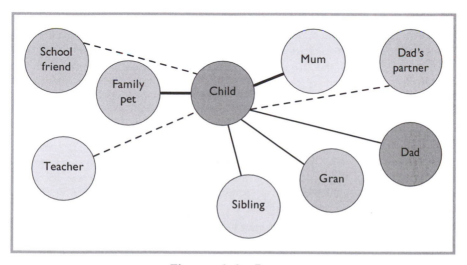

Figure 6.6   Ecomap

Source: Adapted by the authors from an original diagram in Parker and Bradley (2007).

the strength of relationships. Solid lines indicate a strong connection, with dashed ones indicating a more fragile relationship (see Figure 6.6).

Siblings need age appropriate clear information throughout the illness trajectory. Many organizations have dedicated websites for siblings of all ages (see Weblinks box below).

=== **WEB LINKS** ===

Contact a Family	www.cafamily.org.uk
Family Fund	www.familyfund.org.uk
Mencap	www.mencap.org.uk
CLIC Sargent	www.clicsargent.org.uk

Log on to the resources above and find out what is available for siblings of children who require palliative care.

Grandparents

A family assessment will have highlighted the level of involvement grandparents have in family life. Grandparents do not expect to outlive their own children, much less their grandchildren; this is against the natural processes of life and makes grandparents 'secondary observers' (Aldridge 2007: 95) as their (adult) child experiences the pain of losing a child. The effects of critical illness on grandparents has seldom been studied; however, it is imperative for the interdisciplinary team to recognize the active part they often play in family health and illness. Studies from Denmark support this by giving insight into grandmothers' (Hall 2004a) and grandfathers' lived experiences (Hall 2004b) when a small grandchild is critically ill, and a sense of 'double concern' as worry and helplessness in relation to both parent and child is felt. Grandparents who are on the periphery of the family observe changes in family life and may be able to be actively involved in the provision of care and practical tasks – for example, keeping the extended family aware of the child's condition. Professionals may need to negotiate the contact/care input and information-sharing between parent and grandparent. The role of grandparents and the other mechanisms of support are included in the case study below. While it is acknowledged that all individuals within the interdisciplinary team provide support, two perspectives are explored here by way of example.

CLINICAL FOCUS

Sally is 3 months old and has spinal muscular atrophy (SMA) Type I. She was discharged home three weeks ago and lives with her parents and three brothers aged 3, 6 and 7 years. Her life expectancy is less than one year.

Sally has been readmitted to hospital with a life-threatening episode resulting in the introduction of night-time bi-level positive airway pressure (BiPAP) ventilation. She has been fed via naso-gastric tube since birth. Sally's family have recently moved to a new house in an unfamiliar neighbourhood. Dad has had to return to work, leaving home early and returning late. Mum is exhausted and stressed about Sally's care, the family's future and about how they will cope, and is feeling very isolated. Mum had hoped to return to her part-time job after six months but feels that this is now unrealistic. Sally's paternal grandmother lives locally but relationships are ambivalent; there is no other extended family. Hospital staff have referred the family for further support to representatives of the community inter-disciplinary team.

INTERDISCIPLINARY INSIGHT

The role of social worker and specialist palliative care nurse in psychosocial support for child and family

Role of social worker	Role of specialist palliative care nurse
Assess Sally's needs in partnership with her parents	
Arrange regular home visits and methods of maintaining contact in negotiation with family	
Liaise with relevant interdisciplinary team members	
Ensure family are aware of relevant support groups and specialist professionals for SMA	
Attend regular interdisciplinary meetings	
Establish a therapeutic working relationship with family	
Carry out pre-bereavement work	
Discuss support options	Assess Sally's nursing care/symptoms and prepare a plan of care addressing these
Undertake a financial assessment	Facilitate discussion regarding concerns.
Provide information and advice regarding relevant benefits and advocate on behalf of family	Advise key worker and interdisciplinary team regarding condition and expected care required
Provide information and advice regarding practical and financial support available from charities	Support and advise family regarding actual and potential nursing interventions Sally has had or may require
Offer parents the opportunity to meet with other families	Advise on benefits of respite care to Sally and family
	Advise regarding specialist respite support available

INTERDISCIPLINARY INSIGHT
Continued

Offer emotional support to parents and siblings individually or as a family group	Refer for respite support (community and away from home) with parents' agreement
Inform families of support services available(statutory and voluntary) and make appropriate referrals and introductions	Arrange appropriate training for staff and ensure they are competent
Provide age-appropriate information for siblings	Introduce family to respite care staff.
Explore ways in which Sally's grandmother could provide support	Liaise with children's hospice staff

Conclusion

The growing numbers of families requiring paediatric palliative care, and the increasing complexity of caring for many children, has increased the need for support mechanisms for both the child and the family. The impact on families of caring for life-limited/life-threatened children is increasingly being recognized in research, policy and practice. Families involved in paediatric palliative care live with the knowledge that their child will die prematurely. While this final outcome cannot be changed, active, timely and appropriate psychosocial support for the whole family can alleviate some of the formidable stresses experienced. The use of frameworks and care pathways, as highlighted in this chapter, go some way towards providing support in a structured way. Evidence in practice following interprofessional debriefing indicates that positive outcomes are achieved when recommendations made in these and similar documents are followed. However, it is important to remember that support must occur in response to the family's wishes at any given time. Working in partnership with children and parents will ensure that support is both timely and appropriate.

Key resources

Redmond, B. and Richardson, V. (2003) Just getting on with it: Exploring the service needs of mothers who care for young children with severe/profound and life-threatening intellectual disability. *Journal of Applied Research in Intellectual Disabilities* **16**: 205–18.

Brett, J. (2004) The journey to accepting support: how parents of profoundly disabled children experience support in their lives. *Paediatric Nursing* **16**: 814–18.

Kerr, L. M., Harrison, M. B., Medves, J., Tranmer, J. E. and Fitch, M. I. (2007)Understanding the supportive care needs of parents of children with cancer: an approach to local needs assessment. *Journal of Pediatric Oncology Nursing* **24**: 279–93.

CHAPTER SUMMARY

■ Psychosocial support is an integral and vital part of paediatric palliative care.

■ A comprehensive and ongoing child- and family-centred assessment, in partnership with the child and family, is key to identifying all aspects of support required.

■ The nature of support is unique to each child's and family's circumstances, and may be emotional, financial or practical.

■ Respite care is vital, and must be offered early by staff who are trusted by the parents and child, and take place in a setting that is responsive to their needs.

■ The needs of siblings, grandparents and the wider family must not be overlooked.

■ Knowledge of available support is a safety net for families, providing emotional reassurance even if the support offered is not taken up at that time.

References

ACT (Association for Children with Life-threatening or Terminal Conditions and their Families) (2003) *Assessment of Children with Life-Limiting Conditions and Their Families. A Guide to Effective Care Planning*. Bristol: ACT.

ACT (Association for Children with Life-threatening or Terminal Conditions and their Families) (2004) *Integrated Multi-Agency Care Pathways for Children with Life-Threatening and Life-Limiting Conditions*. Bristol: ACT.

Aldridge, J. (2007) *Living with a Seriously Ill Child*. London: Sheldon Press.

Beresford, P., Adshead, L. and Croft, S. (2007) *Palliative Care, Social Work and Service Users. Making Life Possible*. London: Jessica Kingsley.

Beresford, B., Rabiee, P. and Sloper, P. (2007) *Priorities and Perceptions of Disabled Children and Young People and Their Parents Regarding Outcomes from Support Services*. York: Social Policy Research Unit.

Bleakley, K. (2008) A qualitative study of parents' perceptions of 'respite care at home' for life-limited and life-threatened children in one Health and Social Services Board. Unpublished MSc dissertation.

Brett, J. (2004) The journey to accepting support: how parents of profoundly disabled children experience support in their lives. *Paediatric Nursing* **16**: 814–18.

Brody, A. C. and Simmons, L. A. (2007) Family resiliency during childhood cancer: the father's perspective. *Journal of Pediatric Oncology Nursing* **24**: 152–65.

Brown, E. (2007) *Supporting the Child and Family in Paediatric Palliative Care*. London: Jessica Kingsley.

Carers UK (2007) *Real Change Not Short Change: Time to Deliver for Carers*. Available at: www.carersuk.org

Cook, P. (1999) *Supporting Sick Children and Their Families*. London: Bailliere Tindall.

Corkin, D., Price, J. and Gillespie, E. (2006) Respite care for children, young people and families are their needs addressed? *International Journal of Palliative Nursing* **12**(9):422–7.

Cowen, P. and Reed, D. (2002) Effects of respite care for children with developmental disabilities: evaluation of an intervention for at risk families. *Public Health Nursing* **19**(4): 272–83.

Damiani, G., Rosenbaum, P., Swinton, M. and Russell, D. (2004) Frequency and determinants of formal respite service use among caregivers of children with cerebral palsy in Ontario. *Child Care, Health and Development* **30**: 77–86.

DfES and DH (Department for Education and Skills and Department of Health (2004) *National Service Framework for Children, Young People and Maternity Services. Disabled Children and Young People and Those with Complex Health Needs*. Available at: www.dh.gov.uk/en/PublicationsandStatistics/Publications/PublicationsPolicyAndGuidance/DH.4089112.

DH (Department of Health) (2000) *Carers and Disabled Children Act*. London: HMSO.

DH, DfEE and Home Office (Department for Children, Schools and Families) (2000) *Framework for the Assessment of Children in Need*. Available at: www.dh.gov.uk/en/Publicationsandstatistics/Publications/PublicationsPolicyAndGuidance/DH_ 4003256

Dobson, B., Middleton, S. and Beardsworth, A. (2001) *The Impact of Childhood Disability on Family Life*. York: Joseph Rowntree Foundation.

Edwards, M. and Davis, H. (1997) *Counselling Children with Chronic Medical Conditions*. Leicester: British Psychological Society.

Hall, E. O. C. (2004a) A Double Concern: Grandmothers' Experiences when a Small Grandchild Is Critically Ill. *Journal of Pediatric Nursing* **19**(1): 61–9.

Hall, E. O. C. (2004b) A Double Concern: Danish Grandfathers' Experiences when a Small Grandchild Is Critically Ill. *Intensive Critical Care Nursing* **20**(1): 14–21.

Hartnick, C., Bissell, C. and Parsons, S. (2003) The impact of pediatric tracheostomy on parental caregiver burden and health status. *Otolaryngeol Head and Neck Surgery* **129**: 1065–9.

Hartrey, L. and Wells, J. S. G. (2003) The meaning of respite care to mothers of children with learning disabilities: two Irish case studies. *Journal of Psychiatric and Mental Health Nursing* **10**: 335–42.

Heaton, J., Noyes, J., Sloper, T. and Shah, R. (2005) Families' experiences of caring for technology-dependent children: a temporal perspective. *Health and Social Care in the Community* **13**(5): 441–50.

Hewitt-Taylor, J. (2008) *Children with Complex and Continuing Health Needs: The Experiences of Children, Families and Care Staff*. London: Jessica Kingsley.

HM Treasury and Department for Education and Skills (2007) *Aiming High for Disabled Children: Better Support for Families*. Available at: www.hm-treasury.gov.uk

Jones, B. (2006) Companionship, control, and compassion: a social work perspective on the needs of children with cancer and their families at the end of life. *Journal of Palliative Medicine* **9**(3): 774–88.

Kerr, L. M., Harrison, M. B., Medves, J., Tranmer, J. E. and Fitch, M. I. (2007) Understanding the supportive care needs of parents of children with cancer: an approach to local needs assessment. *Journal of Pediatric Oncology Nursing* **24**: 279–93.

Kirk, S. and Glendinning, C. (2002) Supporting 'expert' parents – professional support and families caring for a child with complex health care needs in the community. *International Journal of Nursing Studies* **39**: 625–35.

Laverty, H. and Reet, M. (2001) *Planning Care for Children in Respite Settings*. London: Jessica Kingsley.

Martin, T. and Doka, K. (2000) *Men Don't Cry Women Do*. Levittown, PA: Brunner Mazel.

McGrath, P. (2001) Identifying support issues of parents of children with leukaemia. *Cancer Practice* **9**(4): 198–205.

McLeod, J. (2000) *An Introduction to Counselling*, 2nd edn. Buckingham: Open University Press.

McNeilly, P. and Price, J. (2008) Care of the child after death. In Kelsey, J. and McEwing, G. (2008) *Clinical Skills in Child Health Practice*. London: Elsevier.

Mencap (2001) *No Ordinary Life: The Support Needs of Families Caring for Children with Profound and Multiple Learning Difficulties*. London: Mencap.

Mencap (2003) *Breaking Point: A Report on Caring without A Break for Children and Adults with Profound Learning Disabilities*. London: Mencap.

Montagnino, B. and Mauricio, R. (2004) The child with a tracheostomy and gastrostomy: parents' stress and coping in the home – a pilot study. *Pediatric Nursing* **30**(5): 373–82.

Murphy, G. (2001) The technology-dependent child at home. Part 2: The need for respite. *Paediatric Nursing* **13**(8): 24–8.

NICE (National Institute for Health and Clinical Excellence) (2005) *Guidance on Cancer Services. Improving Outcomes in Children and Young People with Cancer: The Manual.* Available at: www. nice.org.uk/nicemedia/pdf/C&YPManual.pdf

Neufeld, S., Query, B. and Drummond, J. E. (2001) Respite care users who have children with chronic conditions: are they getting a break? *Journal of Pediatric Nursing* **16**(4): 234–44.

NICHCY (National Dissemination Center for Children and Youth with Disabilities) (2005) *Respite Care: A Gift of Time.* Available at: http://old.nichcy.org/pubs/outprint/nd12txt.htm; accessed 16 February 2009.

Nicoll, M., Ashworth, M., McNally, L. and Newman, S. (2002) Satisfaction with respite care: a pilot study. *Health and Social Care in the Community* **10**(6): 479–84.

O'Brien, M. E. (2001) 'Living in a House of Cards: Family Experiences with Long-term Childhood Technology Dependence', *Journal of Pediatric Nursing* **16**(1): 13–22.

Olsen, R. and Maslin-Prothero. P. (2001) Dilemmas in the provision of own-home respite support for parents of young children with complex health needs: evidence from an evaluation. *Journal of Advanced Nursing* **34**(5): 603–10.

OPSI (Office of Public Sector Information) (2001) *Health and Social Care Act.* Available at: www. opsi.gov.uk/acts/acts2001

Parker, D., Maddocks, I. and Stern, L. (1999) The role of palliative care in advanced muscular dystrophy and spinal muscular atrophy. *Journal of Paediatrics and Child Health* **35**: 245–50.

Parker, J. and Bradley, G. (2007) *Social Work Practice: Assessment, Planning, Intervention and Review*, 2nd edn. Exeter: Learning Matters Ltd.

RCN (Royal College of Nursing) (2005) *Memorandum to the Commons Health Committee inquiry into palliative care services.* Available at: www.rcn.org.uk

Redmond, B. and Richardson, V. (2003) Just getting on with it: exploring the service needs of mothers who care for young children with severe/profound and life-threatening intellectual disability. *Journal of Applied Research in Intellectual Disabilities* **16**: 205–18.

Robinson, C., Jackson, P. and Townsley, R. (2001) Short breaks for families caring for a disabled child with complex health needs. *Child & Family Social Work* **6**(1) 67–75.

Rogers, C. G. (1951) *Client-centred Therapy.* Boston, MA: Houghton Mifflin.

SCN (Shared Care Network) (2003) '*Too Disabled for Care?' Report on Short Break Care Services for Children with Complex Health Care Needs.* Available at: www.sharedcarenetwork.org.uk

Steele, R. (2005) Strategies used by families to navigate uncharted territory when a child is dying. *Journal of Palliative Care* **21**(2): 103–11.

Thurgate, C. (2004) Home from home: evaluation of a respite service in Kent. *Paediatric Nursing* **16**(7): 20–2.

Valkinier, B. J., Hayes, V. E. and McElheran, P. J. (2002) Mothers' Perspectives of an In-home Nursing Respite Service: Coping and Control. *Canadian Journal of Nursing Research* **34**(1): 87–109.

Weightman, G. (2000) *A Real Break. A Guidebook for Good Practice in the Provision of Short-Term Breaks as a Support for Care in the Community.* Department of Health. Available at: www.carers.gov.uk

While, A., Citrone, C. and Cornish, J. (1996) *A Study of the Needs and Provisions for Families Caring for Children Living with Life-Limiting Incurable Disorders.* London: Department of Nursing Studies, Kings College Hospital.

Reflection – Advancing Care and Practice

*Patricia McNeilly and Jayne Price**

Introduction

As discussed in Chapter 1, children requiring palliative care represent a diverse group whose illnesses are often prolonged and unpredictable, and this creates many challenges and much stress for children themselves, their families and the professionals who support them (Price and McFarlane 2006). As palliative care for children is a developing area of practice, a commitment by professionals to enhance the evidence base underpinning care delivery has never been greater. While substantiative research around the needs of children and families continues to increase, the experiences of professionals working within the field are also crucial to satisfy current governance arrangements. One method of examining such experiences in a structured way is by means of the process of reflection. As in other areas, reflection in palliative care is concerned with learning that has an impact on future behaviour or professional practice, and engaging in reflection can help to unravel the complexities of working with these particular children and families. It is generally agreed across disciplines that reflecting on practice, both on a personal level or as a team, is one way of improving the care of children and families, and developing services that are responsive and timely. The development and use of reflection as a concept is recounted substantially elsewhere and is therefore not duplicated here; however, interested readers are referred to the key resources at the end of this chapter.

---

* This chapter is reproduced in part from the following article: McNeilly, P., Price, J. and McCloskey, S. (2006) A model for reflection in children's palliative care. *European Journal of Palliative Care* **13**(1): 31–4, with the kind permission of the *European Journal of Palliative Care*.

One way of facilitating reflective thinking and practice is by the use of models as frameworks and a number of these have been developed over recent years (for example, Borton, 1970, Gibbs, 1988, Johns 1995, 2000) and used in a variety of settings. However, the need to adapt present models or frameworks for palliative care has also been demonstrated (see, for example, Souter 2003). The purpose of this chapter is to describe and demonstrate the use of a specific reflective model developed by McNeilly *et al.* (2006) for use by practitioners caring for children requiring palliative care and their families. An example of how the model may be used is included at the end of the chapter.

KEY POINT

Reflection is concerned with learning that has an impact on future behaviour or professional practice.

Why reflect?

Throughout this book, the complexities and challenges of working with children and families requiring palliative care have come to the fore. Professional bodies and educationalists continue to promote reflection as a useful strategy in order to shape future practice, to engender positive coping mechanisms, and to encourage practitioners to question their practice and engage in life-long learning. Reasons why this is particularly important for practitioners working in this field are set out in Figure 7.1. Whether conducted on a personal level, shared in a group situation

---

Requisite – Many professional bodies promote reflection as a requisite skill for entry to the health care professions.

Education – Reflection is a useful strategy to employ in palliative care education, to link theory and practice and encourage practitioners to think critically.

Future practice – Central to reflection is its potential to improve future practice.

Learning – Reflection provides one way of promoting life-long learning and critical thinking skills.

Ethical decision-making – Reflecting in paediatric palliative care may assist with complex ethical decisions.

Catharsis – Reflection may provide opportunities for catharsis and engender ways of coping when faced with stressful situations.

Team debriefing – Group reflection may enhance both team-working and outcomes for children and families.

Figure 7.1   Reasons why reflection is important in paediatric palliative care

or during team debriefing, reflection can serve as a form of catharsis and engender coping mechanisms for those working within this speciality. The challenges of team-working in this area are discussed in Chapter 2, with the need for co-operation highlighted. Clearly, such co-operation may be enhanced by sharing experiences and discussing the performance of the team by reflecting on practice. Similarly, reflecting on experiences concerning communication with the child and family, the management of ethical issues and caring for dying children and their families, as discussed in other chapters, is crucial if services are to continue to be strengthened and further developed.

A model of reflection for use in children's palliative care

As with previous frameworks, the model proposed here (illustrated in Figures 7.2 and 7.3) comprises a series of phases, including a preliminary and a post-reflection phase, and is to some extent influenced by the palliative care model of reflection by Souter (2003) and Johns' model of structured reflection (2000). While the model may at first appear rather complex, only relevant components need to be

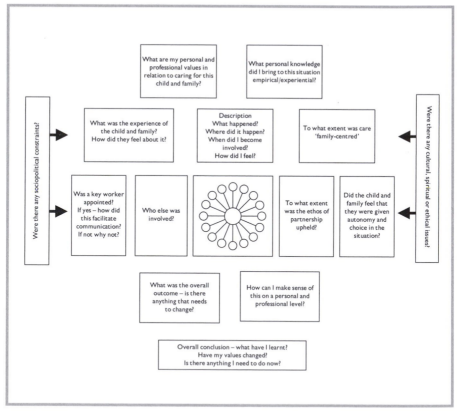

Figure 7.2   A model of reflection for children's palliative care

Source: McNeilly *et al.* (2006).

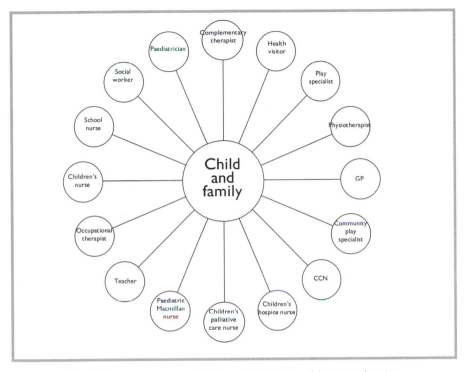

Note: This represents an example of those who may be involved, but is not exhaustive.

Figure 7.3 A model of reflection for children's palliative care

Source: McNeilly et al. (2006).

addressed. For example, reflecting on the role of the key worker may be less relevant in the hospital setting, while ethical issues may be more important for those reflecting on truth telling. Similarly, some more complex situations will warrant the examination of many issues within each phase, while others may be more straightforward but no less important. The following sections describe the different phases of the model.

Preliminary phase

Atkins (2004) highlights the importance of considering one's values when reflecting on practice. This model first challenges practitioners to examine their values in relation to caring for children with palliative care needs and their families (see Figure 7.4). Essentially, values are concerned with what is most important to the practitioner in a given situation; for example, that the child and family receive the highest standard of care, or that the family's wishes are paramount at all times. Also, prior to the first phase of the model, practitioners are required to reflect on their personal knowledge of children's palliative care. This knowledge may come from two sources: experiential knowledge and empirical knowledge. Experiential knowledge arises as a result of having previous experience of a specific situation or

<table>
<tr><td>What are my personal and professional values in relation to caring for this child and family?</td><td>What personal knowledge did I bring to this situation empirical/ experiential?</td></tr>
</table>

Figure 7.4   Preliminary stage

Source: McNeilly *et al.* (2006).

challenge, while empirical knowledge refers to prior learning in terms of relevant training, study or reading. For example, a practitioner may be recently qualified or may have many years of experience in caring for children and families in this situation. Similarly, they may have no additional training or they may have completed in-service or accredited training in this area or acquired knowledge based on their own reading or continuing professional development. Acknowledging empirical and experiential knowledge is important as it frequently has an impact on how one thinks about a given situation.

Phase I – the deductive phase

In keeping with alternative models of reflection, the first phase is concerned with a comprehensive description of events and the cognitions around this (see Figure 7.5). Also considered here are the child and family's perspectives and the extent to which the care was 'family centred'. Throughout the course of this text, the importance of the family in the child's journey is repeatedly highlighted as critical. This is alongside the need for the family to be supported by an interdisciplinary team with the professional knowledge and skills to negotiate with them their desired level of participation in the child's care. Family-centred care has been

<table>
<tr><td>What was the experience of the child and family? How did they feel about it?</td><td>Description What happened? Where did it happen? When did I become involved? How did I feel?</td><td>To what extent was care 'family-centred'</td></tr>
</table>

Figure 7.5   Phase I

Source: McNeilly *et al.* (2006).

described as 'professional support for the child and family through a process of involvement, participation, and partnership, underpinned by negotiation and empowerment' (Smith *et al.* 2002: 22) and this approach has been endorsed by numerous professional and policy documents (Royal College of Nursing 2003, DfES and DH 2004, DH 2007, DH 2008). Caring for a child with a life-limiting illness can have a serious impact on families and on family life (Steele and Davies, 2006) and therefore care that embraces the whole family is essential (Friedman *et al.* 2005). Clearly a comprehensive understanding of the experience as expressed by the child and family is a fundamental part of reflection and the provision of optimal care.

Phase 2

The importance of effective communication has been discussed in many chapters of this text. Consistent with this, the second phase of the model (see Figure 7.6) focuses on two aspects of communication: interdisciplinary working and the associated control experienced by the family in terms of partnership working and their perception of autonomy and choice. Service providers also need to work in partnership and communicate effectively with the help of the key worker. Figure 7.3 shows an example of professionals who may be involved with a child who requires palliative care, making successful communication a challenging issue, as highlighted in Chapters 2 and 3. Numerous researchers have identified the impact of well co-ordinated services on family and parent–professional relationships, quality of life and their satisfaction with services (Beresford 1995, Townsley *et al.* 2004) and so is included in this phase.

The central ethos of true partnership working concerns empowering the family to make informed decisions about their treatment and care. If such autonomy is to be upheld, then clear, concise information is essential (Brown 2002; Price 2003). This can be difficult to achieve, as children with palliative care needs vary in their stages of cognitive development and ability (Hynson *et al.* 2003). Therefore health care professionals must be aware of the stages of child development and potential for regressive behaviour caused by ongoing ill health (Price 2003). When dealing with children with significant cognitive impairment, the

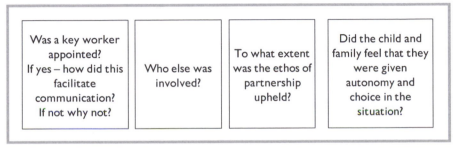

Figure 7.6 Phase 2

What was the overall outcome – is there anything that needs to change?	How can I make sense of this on a personal and professional level?

Figure 7.7 Phase 3

Source: McNeilly et al. (2006).

practitioner is particularly reliant on the judgement and advice of the child's parents or carers.

Clearly, therefore, the complexities around communication, partnership working and the relationship between the team, child and family need careful consideration. This is exactly why they are the cornerstone of quality care, and important within the reflective process.

Phase 3 – the inductive phase

The final phase of the model considers the overall outcome of the reflective process and the identification of the need for change if required. Alternatively, if there has been a positive outcome, it may be beneficial to disseminate good practice to colleagues who work in this field. Given the dearth of research within this arena, this may help to satisfy current governance arrangements in terms of evidence-based practice.

The second element of Phase 3 concerns the notion of sense-making, at both a personal and professional level. According to Ghaye and Lillyman (2000) the process of reflection enables us to make sense of our thoughts and actions in a given situation. Based on the ethos of phenomenology, sense-making acknowledges that routine thinking is at times inadequate, and a new perspective is required so that an individual may move on (Teekman 2000). Given the complex nature of caring for children with life-limiting illness, this would seem to be an appropriate approach. Having broken down an incident into its components parts in the first two phases, this phase gives the practitioner the opportunity to reconstitute it in order to make sense of what has occurred.

Post-reflection phase

The final, or post-reflection, phase involves the formation of an overall conclusion where the practitioner re-examines his or her values and establishes from a personal perspective what has been learnt. This provides an opportunity for personal

Overall conclusion – what have I learnt?
Have my values changed?
Is there anything I need to do now?

Figure 7.8   Post-reflection stage

Source: McNeilly et al. (2006).

growth and continued professional development. It is at this stage that the practitioner may be in a position to apply the outcome of his/her reflection to future practice, to enhance the delivery of palliative care. The individual may also be able to identify any further action that is required; for example, the formation of an interprofessional or user group to examine a particular issue, the need for a research study or the need to provide follow-up care for the child and family. This is perhaps the most important stage.

The Clinical Focus box below demonstrates the use of the model. It describes a reflection by a Ward Manager of a busy neonatal unit around the care of Emma, a baby born with Edwards syndrome, and interaction with her parents.

CLINICAL FOCUS

Emma, a 2-week-old infant, was born at 38 weeks' gestation via caesarian section. She is the first baby of Christine and Michael, both mature parents who previously have experienced a number of miscarriages. During the pregnancy, Emma's parents were very anxious given their past history, but were reassured and while the baby appeared small, no abnormalities were detected. At birth it became immediately apparent that Emma had respiratory difficulties and was noted to have clenched hands and webbing of the second and third toes. A diagnosis of Edwards Syndrome was made and the severity of the situation was explained to Christine and Michael. Currently, she is being cared for in the regional special care baby unit where she is on CPAP because of respiratory difficulties and cardiac abnormalities. Over the past two weeks Christine has become increasingly withdrawn from staff, and Michael in particular has been verbally aggressive to medical and nursing staff on a number of occasions.

McNeilly *et al.* (2006) Model of reflection	Reflection on practice by Simon (Ward Manager)
Preliminary phase Prompts the professional to ask: What are my personal and professional values in relation to caring for this child and family? What personal knowledge did I bring to this situation empirical/experiential?	Simon felt that, for him, one of the most important aspects of working in the neonatal unit was the need to communicate openly and honestly with parents, particularly those who were faced with difficult and emotional situations. As Ward Manager he was also very aware that he was ultimately responsible for the care that infants and their families received, as well as providing support to staff working in this busy and at times stressful unit. Over the years, Simon had encountered many situations where parents struggled to accept the diagnosis and prognosis of their child, and while each situation was different, the current situation was not new to him. Simon had also kept himself up to date in terms of management courses and reading professional journals that discussed parents' experiences of having a child with a life-limiting condition, and ways to support them on their journey.
Phase I – Deductive phase Prompts the professional to ask: What was the experience of the child and family? How did they feel about it? Description of event. What happened? Where did it happen? When did I become involved? And how did I feel? To what extent was care 'family-centred'?	It was becoming increasingly apparent that Emma's parents were finding it desperately hard to cope. They had since Emma's birth become more distant from staff and at times hostile. On a number of occasions, Michael had been verbally abusive to medical and nursing staff and his latest outburst had prompted Simon to call security as he felt that Michael's behaviour was a threat to staff and was clearly upsetting for the other parents on the unit. While Simon understood Michael's behaviour, it was upsetting for everyone involved and in the current atmosphere made it difficult to provide Emma with the care that she needed. The situation was also reducing the ability of staff to provide care that was family-centred, for while every effort was made to encourage the parents to participate as partners in Emma's care and to be involved in decision-making, the lack of communication was creating a barrier to this process. Furthermore, it was difficult to assess exactly how the parents felt about it. It was clear that they were very unhappy, but the current state of the therapeutic relationship was not conducive to sharing their feelings in any detail.

→

Phase 2 – Deductive phase

Prompts the professional to ask:

Was a key worker appointed? If yes:

How did this facilitate communication?

If not, why not? Who else was involved?

To what extent was the ethos of partnership upheld?

Did the child and family feel that they were given autonomy and choice in the situation?

Despite the difficulties concerning partnership, Simon was aware that staff across numerous disciplines were doing their best to involve the parents at all stages in different levels of care and decision-making. Despite the parents being given appropriate information to exercise choice and control over treatment options, they were unable to change the fact that Emma had a serious, life-limiting condition that would require ongoing care. This appeared to make the parents feel powerless, since they were unable to 'fix' Emma's health deficits. Michael had particular anger around the fact that Emma's condition had not been detected ante-natally.

Phase 3 – The inductive phase

Prompts the professional to ask:

What was the overall outcome and is there anything that needs to change?

How can I make sense of this on a personal and professional level?

In the weeks that followed, Simon met the parents regularly to provide support and to reassure them that staff in the unit appreciated they were trying hard to come to terms with their daughter's diagnosis. They were also encouraged to discuss openly any issues they had with Emma's care and participate in decision-making and aspects of her care that they felt were appropriate. Simon set up a meeting with Emma's consultant, who discussed with them their concerns about Emma's diagnosis and the difficulties around the diagnosis. While the relationship between the parents and staff was not optimal, the situation improved and lines of communication were re-established to some degree. It became evident that Michael and Christine were having great difficulty in accepting the situation and forming a bond with their daughter, who they had waited a long time for. While Simon felt that the situation had been handled satisfactorily, on reflection he did feel that earlier intervention, from the time of admission, could have prevented the situation from reaching such a critical level. It also provided a reminder of the many different ways parents react to having a life-limited child, and the need for professionals and others to avoid making judgements and continue to support the family even when it proves difficult.

Post-reflection phase Overall conclusion – what have I learnt? Have my values changed? Is there anything I need to do now?	On reflection, Simon's values had not changed in terms of communicating openly and honestly with parents in the unit, but they had been strengthened. As a manager, he identified a number of issues for action. First, given the differing levels of skill mix and experience of staff in the unit, Simon felt it important to facilitate a structured debriefing session to tease out what he and the team had learnt from this difficult situation that arose while caring. From this session he was able to identify their training needs around the management of difficult situations and bereavement that often starts at diagnosis. Finally, he decided to conduct an audit of parents' experiences within the unit in order to gain further insight into parents' perspectives, including the experiences of fathers, whose views are often overlooked.
Additional elements Socio-political constraints. Cultural/spiritual/ethical issues.	It became evident during the following weeks that Michael and Christine were having great difficulty around spiritual aspects of Emma's birth. They found it difficult to understand why this had happened to them and to Emma, especially since their daughter was much wanted and they had done everything to ensure that they would have a 'healthy' child. Discussions with the hospital chaplain at their request provided some support around the spiritual aspect of their experience.

Additional elements

A number of additional issues arise within the field of palliative care, specifically socio-political constraints and cultural, spiritual or ethical issues. As demonstrated in the Clinical Focus, they warrant consideration when reflecting on practice.

Socio-political constraints

As White (1995) points out, it is imperative that ways of knowing (and indeed the care of children and their families) takes place within the wider context of the socio-political environment. The sociological aspect of the current model recognizes the importance of quality of life and coping mechanisms in families who are already challenged by their social situation.

Political constraints may also have an impact on the provision of care in terms of the constraints of geographical or interagency boundaries, and the model of service provision provided in a particular location. Organizational constraints for example, resource issues may also be an issue depending on the importance attached to paediatric palliative care as a developing area of professional practice.

Cultural/spiritual/ethical issues

The model also takes into account the cultural, spiritual and ethical issues that may have an impact on the situation. Given the increasing multicultural nature of our society, it is imperative that health care professionals develop their existing knowledge about the ethos and practices of different cultures. Indeed, this is essential when fostering the therapeutic relationship with the child and family that is so vital in this domain of practice (Hawes 2005). Spiritual and ethical issues are an inevitable part of caring for life-limited children and are also included. As we have seen in Chapters 4 and 5, they are perhaps one of the most challenging aspects of reflecting on the care of these children and young people, and have been included to some degree in at least one previous model of reflection in palliative care (see Souter 2003).

=== **ACTIVITY** ===

Consider a situation that caused you much thought, or a particular incident that has arisen. Use the model of reflection described here to examine what happened. Is there anything you need to do now?

Conclusion

It is generally accepted across many disciplines that reflecting on practice can, if conducted in a structured manner, potentially improve the quality of care provided in partnership with the child and family. Given the complexity of many aspects of paediatric palliative care, such an approach is further warranted. Using models of reflection can provide a framework for reflective activities, and a specific model for use within this speciality has been presented here. Used on an individual, group or interdisciplinary basis, it is anticipated that the use of this model could encourage discussion and mutual support between practitioners working in this field. Furthermore, it is anticipated that the use of this model could enhance the care of children and families while making an important contribution to the future development of children's palliative care. The concluding chapter of this text will elaborate on other initiatives that will contribute and shape the future direction of care for children with palliative care needs and their families.

Key resources

McNeilly, P., Price, J. and McCloskey, S. (2006) Reflection in children's palliative care: a model. *European Journal of Palliative Care* **13**(1): 31–4.

Rolfe, G., Freshwater, D. and Jasper, M. (2001) *Critical Reflection for Nursing and the Helping Professions*. Basingstoke: Palgrave.

Taylor, B. J. (2006) *Reflective Practice. A Guide for Nurses and Midwives*, 2nd edn. Buckingham: Open University Press.

CHAPTER SUMMARY

▣ Reflection has been used in health care for many years.

▣ Reflection may assist the practitioner with complex and ethical decision-making.

▣ Personal or group reflection may serve as a form of catharsis and help the practitioner to develop coping mechanisms in order to work in this challenging area of practice.

▣ Numerous models of reflection exist; however, a specific model, such as the one presented here, is preferable when reflecting on practice in children's palliative care.

▣ This model may also be used during team debriefing to enhance teamwork at an interdisciplinary and interagency level.

▣ More research is needed in order to demonstrate the benefits of reflection for the practitioner and children and families requiring a palliative approach to care.

Acknowledgement

The author would like to thank Sharon McCloskey, Care Team Manager (Northern Ireland Hospice Care), for her input to the original model and publication.

References

Atkins, S. (2004) Developing underlying skills in the move towards reflective practice. In Bulman, C. and Schutz, S. (eds) *Reflective Practice in Nursing*. Oxford: Blackwell.

Beresford, B. (1995) *Expert Opinions: A Survey of Parents Caring for a Severely Disabled Child*. Bristol: Policy Press.

Borton, T. (1970) *Reach, Teach and Touch*. London: McGraw-Hill.

Brown, E. (2002) *The Death of a Child Care for the Child, Support for the Family*. Birmingham: Acorns Children's Hospice Trust.

DfES and DH (Department for Education and Skills and Department of Health) (2004) *National Service Framework for Children, Young People and Maternity Services*. London: Department of Health.

DH (Department of Health) (2007) *Palliative Care Services for Children and Young People in England. An Independent Review for the Secretary of State for Health*. London: Department of Health.

DH (Department of Health 2008) *Better Care: Better Lives. Improving Outcomes and Experiences for Children, Young People and Their Families Living with Life-Limiting and Life-Threatening Conditions*. London: Department of Health.

Friedman, D., Hilden, J. and Powaski, K. (2005) Issues and challenges in palliative care for children. *Current Pain and Headache Reports* 9: 249–55.

Ghaye, T. and Lillyman, S. (2000) *Reflection: Principles and Practice for Healthcare Professionals*. Dinton: Quay Books.

Gibbs, G. (1988) *Learning By Doing: A Guide to Teaching and Learning Methods*. Oxford: Further Education Unit.

Hawes, R. (2005) Therapeutic relationships with children and families. *Paediatric Nursing* **17**(6): 15–18.

Hynson, J., Gillis, J., Collins, J., Irving, H. and Trethewie, S. (2003) The dying child: how is care different? *Medical Journal of Australia* **179**(6 Suppl): S20–S22.

Johns, C. (1995) Framing learning through reflection within Carper's fundamental ways of knowing in nursing. *Journal of Advanced Nursing* **22**(2): 226–34.

Johns, C. (2000) *Becoming a Reflective Practitioner: A Reflective and Holistic Approach to Clinical Nursing, Practice Development and Clinical Supervision*. Oxford: Blackwell Science.

McNeilly, P., Price, J. and McCloskey, S. (2006) Reflection in children's palliative care: a model. *European Journal of Palliative Care* **13**(1): 31–4.

Price, J. (2003) Information needs of the child with cancer and their family. *Cancer Nursing Practice* **2**(7): 35–8.

Price, J. and McFarlane, M. (2006) Care of the child requiring palliative care. In Glasper, A. and Richardson, J. (eds) *A Textbook of Children's and Young People's Nursing*. London: Elsevier.

RCN (Royal College of Nursing) (2003) *Children and Young People's Nursing: A Philosophy of Care*. London: RCN.

Rolfe, G., Freshwater, D. and Jasper, M. (2001) *Critical Reflection for Nursing and the Helping Professions*. Basingstoke: Palgrave.

Smith, L., Coleman, V. and Bradshaw, M. (2002) *Family-centred Care: Concept, Theory and Practice*. Basingstoke: Palgrave.

Souter, J. (2003) Using a model for structured reflection on palliative care nursing: exploring the challenges raised. *International Journal of Palliative Nursing* **9**(1): 6–12.

Steele, R. and Davies, B.(2006) Impact on parents when a child has a progressive, life-threatening illness. *International Journal of Palliative Nursing* **12**(12): 576–85.

Taylor, B. J. (2006) *Reflective Practice. A Guide for Nurses and Midwives*, 2nd edn. Buckingham: Open University Press.

Teekman, B. (2000) Exploring reflective thinking in nursing practice. *Journal of Advanced Nursing* **31**(5): 1125–35.

Townsley, R., Abbott, D. and Watson, D. (2004) *Making a Difference? Exploring the Impact of Multi-Agency Working on Disabled Children with Complex Care Needs, Their Families and the Professionals Who Support Them*. Bristol: Policy Press.

White, J. (1995) Patterns of knowing: review, critique and update. *Advances in Nursing Science* **17**(4): 73–86.

Symptom Management

Heather McCluggage and Satbir Singh Jassal

Introduction

Effective symptom management is of vital importance to children requiring palliative care, not only to promote comfort but also to enhance quality of life for the child and family (Friedrichsdorf and Collins 2007). Research has demonstrated that unresolved symptoms are not only distressing for children, but can also have a lasting impact on parents for many years afterwards (Frager and Collins 2006). In relation to symptom management in end-of-life care, it would appear that significant progress has been made in recent years. In a US study in 2000, Wolfe *et al.* reported that, according to parents, 89 per cent of children studied suffered 'a great deal' or 'a lot' at the end of life. In a follow-up study (Wolfe *et al.* 2008), children were reported to experience significantly less suffering, and parents were better prepared for the end of life. As with alternative aspects of care discussed throughout this book, successful management of symptoms, whether acute or chronic, is dependent on care that is child-centred and delivered in partnership with the child and parents as experts in their child's care. Furthermore, effective interdisciplinary, interagency team-working (ACT and the RCPCH 2003), in which individuals communicate well with each other, share information, knowledge and expertise across the many disciplines involved, is key to managing children's symptoms. Recent research has investigated the prevalence of symptoms experienced by children at the end of life, with those such as pain, dyspnoea, nausea and vomiting frequently highlighted (Frager and Collins 2006). While the symptoms of children with malignancies or other specific diagnoses are arguably reasonably predictable, symptom profiles of children with complex health needs can be particularly difficult to identify and treat (McCluggage and Elborn 2006). Regardless of diagnosis, it is worth remembering that children are individuals in terms of the way they experience and present with symptoms; what will be distressing to one child may be less so to another. The aim of this chapter is to explore many of these symptoms, from a practical perspective. Research is ongoing and treatments change; however, the basic principles set out in this chapter should not.

A general approach to managing children's symptoms

It has been recognized that caring for a child with palliative care needs can be a stressful experience for parents and carers, the nursing team, the allied health professionals involved and the doctors (Rushton *et al.* 2006). As ACT and RCPCH (2003) point out, individuals working within the field of children's palliative care need to be proficient in the assessment as well as management of symptoms during the course of the child's illness and at the end of life. While a range of assessment tools are available to assist with this process, these are still not widely used in this context. In a recent study of twenty-three children's hospices in the UK, only a quarter of participating doctors and nurses used an assessment tool, and the tools used were specific to pain assessment (McCluggage and Elborn 2006). Regardless of specific techniques, it is worth remembering that the presentation of symptoms represents a complex interplay of physiological, psychological and spiritual factors, not only concerning the child, but also the parents. Using the parents' knowledge of the child combined with close observation probably give the best assessment possible.

Pharmacological management can pose certain challenges within children's palliative care. First, the use of unlicensed drugs is a major concern (Choonara, 2004). As a result, drug use is often extrapolated from adult practice, and doses are based on weight formulas. Furthermore, Hain and Wallace (2008) point out that many of the drugs used in palliative care are not available in oral preparations, or have not been developed for the specific needs of children. They also concede that many children with non–malignant conditions may have some form of enteral feeding device, which may cause inconsistent absorption. While the therapeutic management of symptoms is one of the priorities of research identified by ACT and RCPCH (2003), doing research into the use of palliative care drugs presents major difficulties in terms of ethics and study size because of the small numbers involved (Wong *et al.* 2003). Parents (and appropriately competent children) should always be warned about this whenever treatment with a new drug is started. Parents are very understanding of this provided they are well informed. A number of general principles may be applied in the approach to managing children's symptoms; these are set out in Figure 8.1 below.

It is also important to be prepared for the unexpected. Even those who appear to be following the normal disease pattern may suddenly develop a different symptom from what might be expected. For example, many children with neurological diseases, who normally experience respiratory difficulties, may develop problems with gut motility leading to constipation or ileus. Similarly, the development of stress ulcers with haematemesis, urinary retention or an inability to thermoregulate can all happen suddenly and unexpectedly. Contingency plans must be made for such eventualities.

- Listen to both the child and the parents.

- Work with the parents as experts in their child's care, as some of their more unusual ideas may work.

- Keep it simple.

- Pay close attention to detail.

- Work as a team, hospital, community, hospice.

- Keep all lines of communication open at all times within the team.

- Be supportive of other team members.

- Know your limits and when to ask for help.

Figure 8.1   Principles for effective symptom management

Symptom management for children should combine and integrate both pharmacological and non-pharmacological strategies (Anghelescu *et al.* 2006). It should be recognized that, within the children's palliative care community, complementary and alternative medicine (CAM) is increasingly being used to the great benefit of children and families. While a review of CAM use in children is beyond the scope of this chapter, a number of useful resources have been produced in recent years, for example the national guidelines for the use of CAM therapies in supportive and palliative care (The Prince of Wales's Foundation for Integrated Health and the National Council for Hospice and Specialist Palliative Care Services 2003) and a guide for patients seeking CAM therapies (The Prince's Foundation for Integrated Health 2007). These are not specifically child-focused; nevertheless, they provide detailed information about research into the efficacy of therapies in addition to identifying registered practitioners.

Psychological problems

Children and families encounter psychological as well as physical symptoms in the palliative phase of illness. Parents, in a study by Theunissen *et al.* (2007), indicated that professionals' main focus was on physical symptoms of the child at the exclusion of psychological symptoms. Looking after or being a very ill child carries with it tremendous strain. It is not uncommon to see frustration, fear or guilt coming to the surface. Having the time available to talk these through is of the utmost importance. As discussed in Chapter 3, it is common to see ill children trying to protect their parents, who in turn are trying to protect them. This results in a spiral of non-communication at a time when it is vitally important to say the things that need to be said. The care team can, if not careful, find themselves caught in the midst of truth-telling issues (see Chapters 3 and 4). Involving members of the team such as teachers, chaplains and play therapists may help to facilitate communication between the child and family. There are some specific psychological symptoms that can be helped by the expertise of clinical psychologists or medication if non- pharmacological methods have failed.

Depression

The diagnosis of depression can be difficult in children. Behaviour and expressions of depression are related to developmental stage, external factors such as family, and the disease process. The use of selective serotonin reuptake inhibitors has become very controversial (Hetrick *et al.* 2007). Only Fluoxetine appears not to have been implicated in problems (Emslie *et al.* 2008). It is helpful, if time and resources permit, to involve child psychiatrists and ask them to initiate treatment or therapy. Unfortunately, all treatments take 3–4 weeks to start becoming effective.

Anxiety

The sight of an anxious child is distressing. This can be treated with short-term but fast-acting lorazepam/midazolam, or slower but longer-acting diazepam (Burtles and Astley 1983). Caution needs to be taken with children who have respiratory compromise. In more difficult cases, Methotrimeprazine (O'Neill and Fountain 1999) or chlorpromazine can be used. Sleep disturbance may also be problematic. In the older child, temazepam can be an effective sleeping tablet (Ashton 1994), whereas, in the younger child, antihistamines such as promethazine or drugs such as triclofos can be used. Melatonin is being used increasingly in children with special needs, with excellent results (Zhdanova 2005). However, its use in these cases is unlicensed.

ACTIVITY

Consider who, in your team, is the person best placed to deal with psychological problems.

Seizures

Seizures are frightening episodes to watch, especially if they occur in the palliative phase of an illness in a child who has not had them before. It is important to manage seizures calmly and to give support to those for whom it is a frightening event. Many children with neurodegenerative illnesses will have had seizures of various and varying types from an early stage in their illness, and their parents will be very comfortable in dealing with them. The National Institute for Health and Clinical Excellence (NICE 2004) and good practice suggests the use of monotherapy to treat seizure activity. However, it is not unusual for children with multiple and complex needs to be on multiple anti-epileptic drugs. If a child's seizures suddenly become worse, the cause should be sought. They may be caused by infection (the most common cause), biochemical imbalance, raised intracranial pressure, or hypoglycaemia (Blume 1992). Some children with quite severe epilepsy are managed successfully with a ketogenic diet; however, it is important to remember that these children have no therapeutic safety net if for some reason (usually infection) their ketosis can not be maintained (Prasad *et al.* 1996).

It is important to remember that managing a seizure may mean doing nothing, as many will self-limit within a few seconds or minutes and require no treatment. Many children will not be at all disturbed by absence-type episodes, but the parents may find them quite distressing. The diagnosis of seizure activity can be difficult, and the exclusion of symptoms such as dystonias or choreaform movements, is important (Murphy and Dehkaharghani 1994). If seizures are tonic/clonic in nature, the child is disturbed by the seizure activity or they have potential dangerous consequences (such as variable consciousness during feeding), they should be treated. Children with epilepsy should be under the management of a paediatric neurologist or a paediatrician with a specialist interest.

There are epilepsy syndromes with specific drug regimes for each. Children who develop epilepsy should be investigated thoroughly, though in many children in palliative care, seizure activity is to be expected because of their diagnosis and the progression of the disease.

KEY POINTS

It is important to remember that managing a seizure may mean doing nothing; many will self-limit within a few seconds or minutes and require no treatment.

Persistent seizures

Persistent seizure activity will often respond to buccal midazolam. This mode of administration is more socially acceptable than rectal diazepam, which has been the mainstay of treatment for many years (Scott *et al.* 1999). With ongoing concerns about child protection, especially in vulnerable children, staff of schools and other carers may be willing to be trained to administer buccal midazolam, but feel uncomfortable about rectal diazepam. It is good practice for a test dose of either of these drugs to be given in hospital before they are prescribed for use in the community, as either of them may cause respiratory depression. Occasionally, the effects of buccal midazolam are too short-lived for some children and they respond better to rectal diazepam to deal with prolonged seizures (Camfield 1999). If the child has a nasograstric (NG) or percutaneous endoscopic gastrostomy (PEG) tube *in situ*, diazepam can be easily and effectively administered through it. With either medication, the dose can usually be repeated after 5–10 minutes. In children who do not respond, paraldehyde made up in olive oil can be given rectally. This should be delivered by a glass syringe, but if drawn up and given immediately, a plastic syringe can be used. It has a very powerful smell and is quite irritating to the rectal mucosa. Drugs such as intravenous lorazepam or clonazepam need to be given in a hospital setting as there is a significant risk of respiratory depression.

━━━━━━━━━━━━ **FURTHER READING** ━━━━━━━━━━━━

Read *Newer Drugs for Epilepsy in Children.* Available at:www.nice.org.uk/pdf/ta079 fullguidance.pdf

Towards the end of life, when seizures tend to increase in both frequency and severity, proactive treatment may stop a child going into status. At this stage, oral medication is often a problem, either because of difficulties in swallowing or unpredictable absorption. Decisions then have to be made as to the best treatment options. Midazolam or phenobarbitone can be used subcutaneously and have the advantage of having anxiolytic effects (Grimshaw *et al.* 1995). These drugs usually take over from other oral drugs, but as some of the newer drugs are available in parenteral solution, it may be possible to use these subcutaneously instead of orally. Subcutaneous midazolam may not be just a end-of-life event, and some centres have used subcutaneous drivers for up to four months before death with very good seizure control. It should be remembered that benzodiazepines cause increased secretions in some children, which may have a dose- limiting effect. Anecdotal evidence would suggest that a small dose of diamorphine may reduce the midazolam dose required.

Phenobarbitone has a slower onset of action but a much longer duration of action over 24–72 hours. It can be used very effectively in a syringe driver at the end of life as a replacement for other drugs not easily available in parenteral formulation (Stirling *et al.* 1999). Care must be taken when using phenobarbitone in a syringe driver as it is a very oily solution and does not mix well with other medications. This may necessitate two drivers being erected, but its use can be very worthwhile.

Pain

Pain is one of the most frequently occurring symptoms in children with a life-limiting condition, and as such is often badly managed (Watterson and Hain 2003). It has been identified as the symptom commonly feared by parents (Goldman and Burne 1998). According to (Hunt *et al.* 2003), three forms of knowledge are required for optimal pain assessment and management: knowing the child; familiarity with children with the same or a similar condition; and knowing the science. However, the problem often is in identifying the source of pain. This may be a reflection of the child's age or difficulty with communication in special needs children (see Further Reading, below). However, the simplest and most accurate way to assess a child's pain is to ask the child, the parents, the family and the care team (Twycross *et al.* 1998). Often pain is expressed in terms of behaviour change. A number of pain assessment tools are available for use in a variety of situations and these are listed in Figure 8.2.

- Visual analogue scales – horizontal or vertical; for example, pain ladder, pain thermometer
- Numerical rating scales
- Faces rating scale (Wong and Baker 1998)
- Poker chip
- Eland colour scales
- FLACC
- Riley infant pain assessment scale
- DEWCE
- Paediatric pain profile
- Behaviour checklist by Breau et al. 2001

Figure 8.2 Pain assessment tools for use in children's palliative care

FURTHER READING

Read Dowling, M. (2004) Pain assessment in children with neurological impairment. *Paediatric Nursing* 16(3): 37–8.

Consider the advantages and difficulties of using pain assessment tools with these children.

Following a logical process of pain management can improve the quality of life for a child significantly. An understanding of the underlying disease process may help to identify the source and nature of the pain. It is important to evaluate the cause of pain (see Figure 8.3) as there are some therapeutic pit falls to be avoided; for example, giving morphine for direct visceral involvement pain may make retention of urine or constipation worse. Treatments for specific pains may overlap; for example, adjuvant therapies for neuropathic pain are the recommended treatments, but morphine can also be very effective.

Managing children's pain

The World Health Organization's (WHO's) pain ladder (see Figure 8.4), consisting of a number of incremental steps, is the most widely accepted and frequently used pharmacological approach to pain management in children (Michelson and Steinhorn 2007). The first step includes the use of paracetamol, which is calculated according to the child's weight and given regularly, rather than waiting for the child to present with pain. If this is ineffective, a move up the ladder to the weak opioids, such as codeine or tramadol, is indicated. This can be given as pure codeine or mixed with paracetamol. If this is not effective, there is no benefit in

- Direct visceral involvement

- Bone involvement

- Soft tissue infiltration

- Nerve compression

- Nerve destruction

- Raised intracranial pressure

- Muscle spasm

- Colic/constipation

- Gastritis

- Retention of urine

- Psychological

Figure 8.3   Causes of pain or perception of pain

Source: Reproduced with the kind permission of *The Rainbows Children's Hospice Guidelines* (Jassal, 2008).

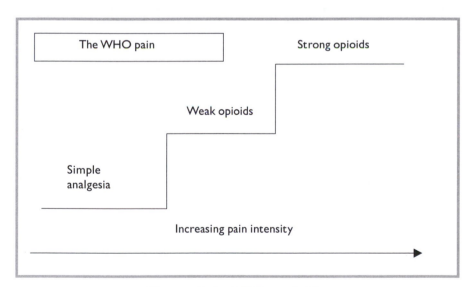

Figure 8.4   WHO pain ladder

Source: World Health Organization (1998). Reproduced with the kind permission from WHO, Cancer Pain Relief and Palliative Care in Children.

trying all the different types of weak opioids; it is always better to move up the ladder and commence a strong opioid, such as morphine. There is often hesitancy in progressing to strong opioids when weak opioids are ineffective, which appears to be around concerns related to morphine. The use of morphine carries many myths, such as 'it shortens life', 'it is the beginning of the end', 'and the child will get addicted to it' (Brown 2007). These misconceptions can result in a barrier to better pain management for the child (Sourkes *et al.* 2005), therefore it is the responsibility of the care team to dispel these ideas and give the parents an accurate informed opinion to allow them to make the decisions they need to care for their child.

Using morphine

Opioids are identified by Sourkes *et al.* (2005: 374) 'as the cornerstone of therapy for moderate to severe symptoms' in children. Morphine should be started in an oral formulation and given at regular 4–6-hourly intervals. The dose should be calculated according to the child's weight rather than his or her age. The child should then be given additional doses of morphine if breakthrough pain continues. After 24 hours, the total dose of morphine given to the child to control pain should be calculated and then divided into regular doses for the next 24 hours. This process should continue until the child's pain has been controlled and the dose of morphine stabilized. The dose of morphine to control breakthrough pain is one-sixth (1/6) of the total 24-hour dose (Drake and Hain 2006). Once the dose of morphine is stable, it can be converted to slow–release morphine (tablets or granules) and given twice daily. It is important to continue to give the child additional morphine if he or she suffers breakthrough pain. There are now a number of alternatives to morphine such as oxycodone (Czarnecki *et al.* 2004) and hydromorphone (Friedrichsdorf and Kang 2007). As a general rule, it is best to use morphine, as there is really little additional benefit in the use of the others. However, these alternatives may be used if the child is intolerant to morphine, or opioid rotation is required to minimize side effects.

▪ Oral diamorphine and morphine are equipotent.

▪ Peak blood levels of intravenous diamorphine are approximately double that of an s.c. or i.m. dose.

▪ Peak plasma levels of morphine/diamorphine occur approximately 30 minutes after i.m. or s.c. injection, but 2–3 hours after setting up a continuous s.c. infusion.

▪ Subcutaneous injection or infusion of diamorphine is 1.5 times as potent as morphine (for example, 15 mg morphine s.c. = 10 mg diamorphine s.c.).

▪ Oral morphine is only half as potent as by injection.

▪ Thus oral morphine dose conversion to diamorphine subcutaneously or by infusion is one-third (for example, 30 mg morphine p.o. = 10 mg diamorphine s.c.).

Notes: s.c. = subcutaneous; i.m. = intramuscular; p.o. = by mouth.

Figure 8.5 Comparison of morphine and diamorphine

Source: Reproduced with the kind permission of *The Rainbows Children's Hospice Guidelines* (Jassal, 2008).

Using diamorphine

Diamorphine is best used when a child is unable to take oral morphine (Hewitt *et al.* 2008). Because of its solubility, it is a very effective drug when given by intravenous, intramuscular or subcutaneous routes. If it is unavailable, then morphine is a perfectly good substitute, but one must be wary of dose calculations. Figure 8.5 compares the properties of morphine and diamorphine.

Retention of urine can be a problem with opioid use. Occasionally, catheterization is necessary with a small gauge catheter or feeding tube. This may be improved by using carbachol or bethanechol (Durant and Yaksh 1988, Asantila *et al.* 1993), or the use of fentanyl, which causes less fewer problems with retention than others. Fentanyl or buprenorphine patches can be particularly useful in children whose pain control is stable (Hunt *et al.* 2001, Noyes and Irving 2001).

──────────────── **ACTIVITY** ────────────────

What non-drug therapies could be used to help alleviate pain?
What myths about morphine have you come across?

Adjuvant therapy

Adjuvant therapies can be introduced at all levels of the WHO ladder, depending on the nature of the pain:

- NSAIDs, such as ilbuprofen or diclofenac are particularly useful for bone and musculoskeletal pain; however, they can cause gastric irritation and ulcers.

- Steroids are effective in cases of pain from raised intracranial pressure, bone pain and pain from nerve infiltration (Klepstad *et al.* 2005). They have serious side effects in children and are best given in short bursts.

- Antidepressants of the tricyclic family, such as amitriptyline, are effective for neuropathic pains often described as a burning sensation.

- Anticonvulsants such as carbamazepine, sodium valproate or gabapentin are also helpful in neuropathic pain (often described as 'stabbing') (Swerdlow, 1980, Golden *et al.* 2006).

- Antispasmodics such as diazepam or baclofen may also be used and are discussed elsewhere in this chapter.

- Others, such as methadone, ketamine, radiotherapy or, nerve blocks are best left to the specialist pain service.

Spiritual pain

This is something that is often overlooked, but is a major cause of distress and if managed correctly can relieve major distress to the child and family. Often confused with religion (which can represents one major part of it), spiritual pain is pain of the soul and can be manifest in the child or any member of the family. This is further discussed in Chapter 5.

Muscle spasm

Muscle spasm is painful and may occur as a result of epilepsy, poor seating/positioning, or progressive neurological disease. It may also be a response to pain. Distressed or agitated children can become quite calm again as their spasm is treated. Multidisciplinary working to ensure good seating in a secure position to keep the child comfortable is of the utmost importance. Advice to parents on moving and handling may reduce the child's spasm and also minimize any trauma to the carer. Full use of the interdisciplinary team should be made to promote the child's comfort in different settings – home, school and so on (Graham and Robinson 2005).

Baclofen is the usual drug of choice for first-line treatment. Starting with a small dose and working upwards allows parents and professionals to monitor closely the child's response. If the central tone drops, or epilepsy is adversely affected, then the baclofen must be stopped. Slow upward titration also minimizes the central side effect of drowsiness. Several centres around the UK now use baclofen pumps to deliver the dose (Emery 2003, Motta *et al.* 2007). This form of treatment is highly effective in appropriately selected cases.

Diazepam is sometimes useful in those cases where spasticity varies depending on how active the child is and if they are having a difficult day (Mathew *et al.* 2005). It can be used for short courses when necessary. However, the sedating effects and increase in secretions can limit its use. Other possibilities are dantrolene (Drake and Hain 2006) and tizanidine (Wallace 1994). As with many drugs used in this context, these are used outside of a product licence and therefore are better under the instruction of a paediatric neurologist.

Nausea and vomiting

The mechanism of nausea is an intricate one, with physical and psychological inputs each interacting with the other. It is therefore an area where a logical system of treatment will cause the greatest effect. Alongside medication, simple common sense measures such as avoiding known stimuli to vomiting – for example, over-feeding, dislikes, types of texture, smells and so on – may be effective. Pain in itself can cause nausea, as can constipation and cytotoxic drugs (Santucci and Mack 2007). Hypercalcaemia in children with malignancies should be excluded. For drug treatment to be effective it must be aimed at the cause of the nausea/vomiting and the physiological pathway as illustrated in Figure 8.6.

The vomiting centre in the brain receives stimuli from all areas of the body and brain. Vomiting can be caused by one or many stimuli. The art of diagnosis and treatment is to work out the interruption of which pathway will be the most

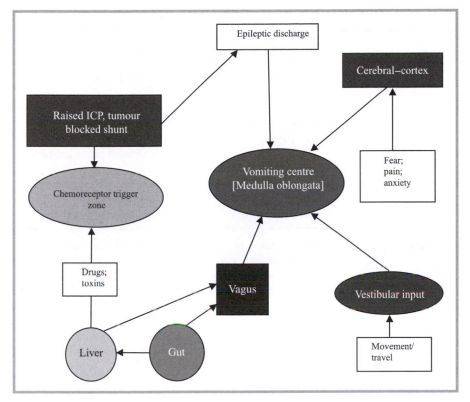

Figure 8.6 Relationship of vomiting centre to stimuli

effective. Drugs that act directly on the chemoreceptor trigger zone or the vomiting centre can be thought of as more broad-spectrum. The use of commonly used anti-emetics is shown in Table 8.1.

Treatment for nausea and vomiting, although readily available, must be administered with care. Giving an already nauseated child oral medicine may cause retching. If gastric stasis is part of the problem, absorption may be delayed. Children who are actively vomiting cannot be given anti-emetics orally. The administration of drugs has become easier, as many are available either as PR, buccal or 'melt' formulations, thus avoiding the intramuscular route. In end-stage care, an anti-emetic can be added to the drugs used for seizure or pain control and given subcutaneously by syringe driver.

Gastro-oesophageal reflux

This is very common, being seen in 50 per cent of neurologically impaired children (Ceriati *et al.* 2006). The most common presentations are refusal to feed, increased respiratory secretions, aspiration pneumonia/recurrent chest infections

Table 8.1   Site of action of anti-emetic drugs

Drug	Site of action	Notes
Haloperidol	Chemoreceptor trigger zone	Anxiolytic benefits
Thioridazine	Chemoreceptor trigger zone	May have some benefits in epilepsy, although generally phenothiazine can exacerbate epilepsy
Chlorpromazine	Chemoreceptor trigger zone	Sedation benefits Contra-indicated in epilepsy
Prochlorperazine	Vestibular centre and Chemoreceptor trigger zone	Side-effects in children limit use
Ondansetron	Chemoreceptor trigger zone Medulla oblongata May also work at vagal level	Side-effects of flushing, headaches and constipation More effective combined with corticosteroids (dexamethasone) Onset of action 30 mins; peak 1–2 hrs; duration 12 hrs
Cyclizine	Medulla oblongata	Commonly used and highly effective Sedating antihistamine with antimuscarinic properties May crystallize with diamorphine in subcutaneous infusion Side-effects drowsiness, dry mouth, blurred vision, urinary retention Onset 30 mins; peak 2 hrs; duration 4–6 hrs
Levomepromazine	Effects at all levels	Phenothiazine Broad spectrum Use when there is failure of specific anti-emetic Stable with diamorphine in subcutaneous infusion Side-effects sedative and postural hypotension

Table 8.1 Continued

Drug	Site of action	Notes
Domperidone	Vagal sympathetic	Prokinetic in upper gut Good for dysmotility in neurological conditions
Metoclopramide	Vagal sympathetic	Crosses blood/brain barrier Causes extrapyramidal side-effects in children; limit use
Dexamethasone	Intracranial pressure	Use in short bursts because of side-effects Reduces permeability of chemoreceptor trigger zone and blood/brain barrier to emetogenic substances and reduces GABA in brainstem

Source: Reproduced with the kind permission of *The Rainbows Children's Hospice Guidelines* (Jassal 2008).

and irritability (Salvatore and Vandenplas 2003, Gold, 2004, Salvatore *et al.* 2004). Other presentations include:

- Vomiting (especially at the end of or after feeds, or when lying flat)
- Difficulty in swallowing
- Haematemesis/melaena
- Cough/wheeze/choking
- Weight loss/failure to thrive
- Difficulty in feeding characterized by:
  - Hyperextensioning of neck
  - Sandifer syndrome (Lehwald *et al.* 2007) (characterized by neck extension after feeds with iron deficiency anaemia and severe oesophagitis).

Initial treatment involves simple measures, such as dividing the child's daily food intake into smaller, more frequent amounts. Feeds, if liquid, can be thickened with gum or starch. Care needs to be taken to ensure that a child fed by nasogastric (NG) tube is not overfed, as this can make the symptoms worse. Positioning during feeding is important; the child should be fed sitting up and kept in an upright position for at least an hour after a feed. Only after these simple measures fail should drug treatment be considered. Antacids can be used with good effect; for example, Gaviscon neutralizes acid and causes a float to protect the oesophagus from refluxing acid. H2 antagonists such as ranitidine would be considered second-line in gastro-oesophageal reflux but certainly have a place prophylactically for children who are taking NSAIDs for pain, to prevent gastric ulceration. One of the mainstays of treatment is proton pump inhibition, either orally or enterally. For administration by NG tube, omeprazole MUP formulation dispersed in a large volume of water or dissolved in sodium bicarbonate can be used. Lansoprazole fastabs can be dissolved in water.

Prokinetic drugs such as Motilium can also be used to empty the stomach contents faster, so less is available to reflux (Keady 2007). Surgical treatment, usually fundoplication and/or pyloroplasty (Bais *et al.* 2000), should only be considered if weight loss or symptoms persist. This can often be performed at the same time as PEG tube insertion. The risks of anaesthesia have to be taken into consideration and post- operative problems are common (25–50 per cent). However, the operation is effective in over 80 per cent of cases.

KEY POINT

Think simple. Try common-sense measures first. And be led by what the parent feels will work best.

Constipation

The process of defecation is both a physical and a psychological one. Chronic constipation in children can be caused by environmental factors just as easily as dietary or medical ones. When dealing with the child in palliative care, all possible causes of constipation should be explored before treatment is begun. Issues for consideration are highlighted in Figure 8.7.

The answers to the questions in Figure 8.7 allow common- sense steps to be taken to promote better bowel control. As with the management of other symptoms discussed in this chapter, an interdisciplinary approach is paramount. Psychological and social issues may need to be addressed with the child, parents and possibly the teacher. Adaptations to allow easier toileting may need to be provided by OT services, and alterations in the diet as recommended by the dietician may be needed to increase fluid or fibre, either by fruit or vegetables or, if PEG or NG fed, by changing the prescribed feed (for example, Nutrini to Nutrini fibre).

Abdominal examination may reveal a sausage-shaped mass in the left iliac fossa or the descending colon. Rectal examination should only be performed if necessary to see if the rectum is empty, (high impaction), full of hard stool (low impaction), or full of soft stool. Impaction may present with watery overflow stool being mistaken for diarrhoea. The use of a glycerine suppository should help the child distressed by constipation when the rectum is full of hard stool. If the stool is soft, a bisacodyl suppository should encourage evacuation, and if the rectum is empty, either a bisacodyl suppository or a phosphate enema is often effective. If the suppositories are not enough to stimulate evacuation, then a MicraLax enema may have to be used.

1. The disease process:
   - Is constipation expected as part of the disease?
   - Is the child an oncology patient?
   - Is dehydration expected because of anorexia?
   - Hypercalcaemia or hypokalaemia?
   - Is the child immobile because of a neurological disorder?
   - Is the child's neurodegenerative condition likely to affect gut enervation and make constipation more likely?
   - Does the child have cystic fibrosis?
   - What is the child's food intake like?

2. Psychological issues:
   - Has the child had a previous episode of constipation that has left them fearful of causing pain by passing stool again?
   - Possibility of rectal tears in this situation?
   - Does the child have a fear of going to the toilet away from home, or with a carer rather than parent.

3. Social/environmental issues:
   - Are there appropriate toilet facilities?
   - Especially in school setting or away from home?
   - Is the child able to ask to use the toilet?

4. Drugs:
   - Is the child on any drugs that might cause constipation? (Opioids, anticholinergics, anticonvulsants, some antibiotics)
   - If the child has been prescribed laxatives, are they being taken?

Figure 8.7   Issues for consideration in the treatment of constipation

The use of rectal preparations should be reserved for those children who are distressed and for whom it is felt immediate relief is required. It is unpleasant to be given an enema, both in the administering and in the effects. Therefore, if the child is not distressed but impacted, clearing with Movicol (see British National Formulary for Children, (2008) for schedule) is preferable and the dose can be titrated as maintenance therapy (Pashankar and Bishop 2001, Candy *et al.* 2006, Thomson *et al.* 2007).

If constipation without impaction is present, it has been common practice to start with an osmotic laxative such as lactulose, building up the dose over a few days, adding a stimulant such as senna, co–danthramer or sodium picosulphate if this proves unsuccessful. If the child is on an opioid they should have a stimulant laxative prescribed at the beginning of treatment. Movicol can be used alone. The volume that has to be administered sometimes restricts its use, but it is usually very well tolerated, and very effective (it is licensed for over-2s only, but has been used unlicensed in under-2s). Prokinetics such as metoclopramide (Demol *et al.* 1989), or erythromycin (Bellomo–Brandao *et al.* 2003) can also be used.

Table 8.2 Drugs to treat constipation

Laxative	Route	Onset	Mechanism	Notes
Rectal preps				
Olive/Arachis oil	PR	Within hours	Lubricates by penetrating and softening stool	Beware peanut allergy!
Docusate Sodium	PR	20 min	Increases water penetration into stool	
Phosphate	PR	30 min	Releases water from faeces and stimulates bowel	Can be very effective but biochemical imbalance possible if repeated.
MicraLax	PR	15–30 min	Osmotic effect	Can cause sodium retention in susceptible individuals
Bisacodyl	Sup	20–60 min	Stimulant	Can cause abdominal cramps
Glycerine	Sup	15–45 min	Lubricant and stimulant	Moisten with water before insertion
Oral osmotic				
Lactulose	Oral	36–48 hr	Osmotic retention of water	First line treatment. Liquid very sticky and sweet
Movicol	Oral	24–48 hr	Glycol retains fluid in bowel	Very effective. Volume needed can be a problem
Stimulant laxatives			Increase intestinal motility	
Senna	Oral	8–12 hr		Available in tablet, granule or syrup preparations
Docusate sodium	Oral	1–2 days		Do not give with liquid paraffin
Bisacodyl	Oral	10–12 hr		Not for prolonged use
Co-danthramer	Oral	8–12 hr		Possibly carcinogenic. May turn urine red. Not first-line
Sodium picosulfate	Oral	6–12 hr		Can be used long-term if necessary.

Source: Reproduced with the kind permission of *The Rainbows Children's Hospice Guidelines* (Jassal, 2008).

Prevention is always better than having to treat, though. If the child is likely to suffer from constipation, prophylactic treatment should be started, and *always* if an opioid is added. Commonly used drugs are listed in Table 8.2.

KEY POINT

Prevention is always better than cure. Anticipate possible constipation and avoid it.

Diarrhoea

Faecal impaction should first be considered (and treated if necessary), before other causes such as gastroenteritis, malabsorption, drugs, a gastrointestinal problem such as colitis, or radiotherapy/chemotherapy. Stool cultures may be needed for an accurate diagnosis. As always, simple measures usually work best. Clear fluids only – for example, dioralyte – should be given for 24–48 hours, followed by resumption of NG or PEG feeds at half or full strength, depending on what the child is able to tolerate. Diarrhoea caused by antibiotic therapy may respond to Lactobacillus treatment, via live yoghurt or a similar produce, which can also help with the common subsequent nappy rash. If these simple, non-pharmacological measures are ineffective, drug treatment should be added.

Initial treatment starts with loperamide (Li *et al.* 2007) at the appropriate age-dependant dose with every loose stool. If this treatment fails, then Lomotil (Demol *et al.* 1989) should be tried. In HIV-induced diarrhoea, metronidazole can be very effective.

Cough

Cough is a common symptom in a range of normal childhood illnesses, and the palliative cohort of patients are no exception. The aetiology needs to be determined (see Figure 8.8) followed by active treatment.

Treatment of the underlying cause is always best, but it is not always possible, and symptomatic treatment must start. Simple measures such as physiotherapy with or without postural drainage, correct positioning, and humidified air or nebulized saline may work well. However, treatment with a cough suppressant may be needed, starting with codeine, and progressing to morphine linctus (Duval and Wood 2002). Sub-clinical seizure activity causing coughing may be associated with screaming or retching and tends to be paroxysmal or clustered (Fogarasi *et al.* 2006). This usually occurs in a child who is known to have epilepsy.

Dyspnoea

The frightening feeling of not being able to breathe properly can happen during choking, a coughing spasm or on its own. It can also be associated with psychological symptoms such as anxiety or panic. There are a number of different causes, as

- Infections
- Gastro-oesophageal reflux (GER)
- Cystic fibrosis
- Heart failure
- Lung metastases
- Aspiration caused by swallowing difficulty/problems with secretions
- Seizure activity
- Neurodegenerative disorders
- Drug induced

Figure 8.8   Causes of cough

Sources: Collins et al. (2000), Simonds (2006), Lavy (2007).

- Anaemia
- Anxiety
- Cerebral tumours
- Congenital heart disease
- Cystic fibrosis
- Hepatic or renal failure
- Infection
- Muscle problems/neurodegenerative disorders
- Other metabolic disorders
- Pleural effusions
- Raised intracranial pressure
- Secondary tumours

Figure 8.9   Causes of dyspnoea

Source: Ullrich and Mayer (2007).

illustrated in Figure 8.9. Anything that reduces lung capacity, chest muscle activity, or transfer of oxygen across the membrane can cause dyspnoea.

Calming the situation is very important. Even if there is a good physical reason for the dyspnoea, anxiety can often make the situation worse. Calm reassurance, oxygen if available, or even blowing into a paper bag will all help. Nebulized saline (to break up thick secretions), bronchodilators or analgesics can work well

(Collins and Fitzgerald 2006). Even in the absence of wheeze, nebulized salbutamol or ipratropium can give symptomatic relief. Oral morphine or subcutaneous diamorphine (in half the analgesic dose) may also help (Viola *et al.* 2008) by acting directly on the respiratory centres and reducing pulmonary artery pressure (this effect is more marked with diamorphine). They will also relieve pain and anxiety.

Excessive salivary/respiratory secretions

Many children with cerebral palsy or neurodegenerative conditions have either excessive salivary/respiratory secretions or have difficulty handling their secretions, thus causing drooling. This is usually more distressing for the parents than the child.

Choking on saliva, however, can be both distressing and dangerous. At present, the mainstay of treatment remains the anticholinergics (Van der Burg *et al.* 2006). The vast majority of children will benefit from the use of a hyoscine hydrobromide patch (Tscheng 2002). If there is concern about tolerability, then an oral dose can be given. In end-of-life care, hyoscine can also be used subcutaneously.

If hyoscine is not effective or side-effects restrict its use, glycopyrronium can be tried (Blasco and Stansbury 1996) (outside product licence). Benzodiazepines can cause excessive secretions, and this side-effect may limit their use. Surgery should not be dismissed, but discussed with an ear, nose and throat (ENT) or plastic surgeon. An emerging treatment is an injection of botulinum toxin into the salivary glands (Van der Burg *et al.* 2006). Noisy secretions near the time of death, known as the death rattle, can be very distressing, especially for the parent or carer. This can be treated with diazepam rectally, or diamorphine, midazolam or hyoscine subcutaneously (Jassal 2008). The following case study illustrates how respiratory symptoms can arise as a result of feeding difficulties and aspiration.

CLINICAL FOCUS

Niamh is a 9-year-old girl with Batten's disease. She has been known to Speech and Language Therapy since her original referral to the service with developmental delay. Her condition has recently deteriorated in that she is having difficulty feeding and in particular with managing thin liquids. In her referral it is noted that she has begun to have chest infections.

A formal request for a clinical feeding evaluation was made by her Consultant Paediatrician.

Niamh attends the local special school.

INTERDISCIPLINARY INSIGHT

The role of the Speech and Language Therapist in Niamh's care

- Complete a full feeding history with Niamh's parents and observe her feeding.

- Establish if there is a risk of aspiration.

- Provide feedback to Niamh's parents and recommend referral for videofluoroscopy at regional centre (liaise with paediatrician).

- Discuss videofluoroscopy procedure with Niamh's parents.

- Provide advice to make Niamh's feeding as safe as possible in the meantime.

- Provide report for paediatrician/interdisciplinary team.

- Liaise with regional SLT re: results of videofluoroscopy; update feeding advice as necessary.

- Liaise with school staff about feeding guidelines.

- Review Niamh's feeding as required.

Written by Ursula Sheerin, Speech and Language Therapist.

Other members of the interdisciplinary team will be involved, in partnership with the family, and their roles are listed in the box below.

OTHER DISCIPLINES INVOLVED IN NIAMH'S CARE

Physiotherapist	For posture control and seating.
Occupational therapist	For seating and feeding utensils.
Dietician	To discuss with parents the availability of suitable foods and textures, range of food types with appropriate textures and so on.
Pharmacist	To see what drug formulations are available for Niamh, to improve convenience and compliance.
Community children's nurse	To monitor general health status and ongoing home care.
Paediatrician	To monitor health status, change in medications and so on.
School staff	To monitor feeding in school.

Bleeding

Bleeding is frightening for the child and distressing for the parents, and may occur from any orifice, including the mouth, rectum or bladder. While it is painless, a major haemorrhage can cause the child to panic, and buccal midazolam or rectal diazepam along with a little diamorphine or morphine (buccal or subcutaneous) may calm the situation, reduce panic and make the child's death less traumatic. Slight ooze from gums etc can be treated with gauze soaked in 1:1000 adrenaline, tranexamic acid mouthwash or Gelfoam. The use of tranexamic acid (intravenous solution) instilled down an NG tube or catheter can reduce bleeding from stomach or bladder significantly in the terminal phase, reducing parental distress. Vitamin

K may help in bleeding due to liver dysfunction, although bleeding caused by liver disease or malignancies should be anticipated and managed by the specialist teams involved.

End-of-life care

The care of the child at the end of life is complex (Wolfe *et al.* 2000) and diagnosis of the end-of-life phase can be very difficult. Children with malignant disease usually follow a more predictable pattern at this stage, thus making decisions about syringe drivers and management more straightforward (Houlahan *et al.* 2006).

Parents and professionals, to a certain extent, often feel that a syringe driver equals expected death in the next 48 hours. However, this is not always the case. Indeed, it is the authors' experience that erecting a driver because of difficulty in oral administration of drugs may cause the child to recover enough for the driver to be taken down. A number of additional factors are worth considering when using syringe drivers with children, as highlighted in the recommended reading below.

FURTHER READING

Read McNeilly, P, Price, J. and McCloskey, S. (2004) The use of syringe drivers – a paediatric perspective. *International Journal of Palliative Nursing* 1(8): 399–403.

Consider how the evidence presented in this article might influence your practice.

The preparation for the end of life is vitally important in ensuring a 'good death' (Hinds, Fouladi, *et al.* 2005); see Chapter 9. Parents and carers vary in how ready they are to hear the news that the end of life is approaching. Parents often know themselves, but confirmation of their worst fears is difficult to accept. Many professionals, especially if it is their first experience, will find this time very emotionally draining. Maintaining a professional distance can be difficult to achieve in practice. It is essential to have parents and the care team working together if there are to be no regrets after the child's death. This may require long negotiations about what is wanted and what is feasible (Hinds, Wolfe *et al.* 2005), together with complex decision-making around continued drug interventions. On a more basic level, involving the parents in promoting their child's comfort is especially important at this time. Making a child comfortable by looking after their mouth and skin is one way in which a parent or carer can feel they are having a real input into the child's care, especially in the end stage. A number of problems may arise in relation to mouth and skin care as the child's condition deteriorates. While a discussion of these is beyond the scope of this short chapter, further information is available within the *The Rainbows Hospice Guidelines* (Jassal 2008).

Members of the team should be prepared to sit down with the parents and give an honest opinion on what is likely to happen in the last hours or days, and also to admit that they might get it wrong The parents should be given information about what to do at the time of death and afterwards, as highlighted in Chapter 9, in a format that is appropriate to their culture. They should be warned in advance of any local differences from what is stated. The child and parents should lead the decision-making, while staff keep them informed in a realistic way about possibilities. People face death in individual ways: some will want the company of a health professional near the time of death; others will want to be on their own with their child; and some will want to have extended family with them at home. As far as possible, the family should be allowed to choose the place of death, with as much or as little support as they require or request.

If the child is cared for at home, where support may not be available on a continuous basis, a symptom flowchart may be particularly useful to guide decision-making around the management of symptoms (see Further Reading box below).

FURTHER READING

Read Willis, E (2007) Symptom care flowcharts: a case study. *Paediatric Nursing* **19**(1): 14–17.

Consider how such a flowchart could have been used for a child and family you have cared for.

End-of-life decisions

When the end-of-life phase appears to have been reached, certain decisions have to be made and discussed:

The drug regime

Unnecessary drugs can be discontinued for example, vitamin supplements or drugs for diarrhoea or nausea – if the oral route is no longer being used. The most important drugs to retain are usually:

- for pain;
- for seizure activity; and
- for agitation.

A compromise may be needed, between what is given orally, per rectum, transdermally and subcutaneously. The use of all routes allows more drugs to be given without overloading any one delivery system. Some drug regimes may need to be changed; for example, phenobarbitone in a syringe driver may be used instead of two or three oral anticonvulsants being given.

Feeding

It is a parent's instinct to feed their child and a very difficult decision to stop doing so. If the child is PEG or NG fed, then feeding can be continued as long as necessary, and water may be given when full feeds have stopped. At this stage in the disease, measures to ensure the child's comfort are paramount. Negotiation with the parents may be necessary to find a level of fluid intake that they are happy with, while making sure that the child is neither nauseated nor vomiting. Small regular sips of fluid or small amounts of fluid by NG or PEG (sometimes as small as 5–10 ml per hour) may be enough to keep the child comfortable and minimize dehydration. Again, some children may stop feeding and then improve again for a time, and the parents want to start re-feeding. It is extremely important at this stage that the parents feel they have done their utmost for their child, so an informed decision should be made by them (Whittam 1993, Dyregrov 2004).

Antibiotics for infection

Parents will want their child to be as comfortable as possible during their final days. Most doctors will treat infections with simple oral antibiotics, on the grounds that it might make the child more comfortable; however, the use of intravenous antibiotics is usually considered invasive. Again, this is a decision that has to be made as a team, including the parents, so that regrets are kept to a minimum (Massimo 2001).

The need for a written 'do not resuscitate' order

If the child is dying at home this is usually unnecessary if the parents and all the carers are in agreement that comfort and not cure is the aim of care (see McCallum *et al.* 2000, Lago *et al.* 2007). However, if the child is in hospital, the wishes of the parents (and child if appropriate) may need to be documented. It can be very distressing for a parent, who has agreed that comfort procedures only will be used, to arrive at the hospital to find their child having invasive treatment because the junior staff are uncertain about what to do.

It is important to remember that unless you have lost a child you cannot say to a parent 'I know how you feel': you don't! The importance of allowing time for a professional debrief (Rushton *et al.* 2006) and attendance at funerals and so on, covered in Chapter 10, cannot be overemphasized.

Conclusion

As Goldman *et al.* (2006) point out, the management of symptoms in paediatric palliative care is very much based on the clinical expertise of those involved, and evidence extrapolated from adult palliative care research and literature. Many of the studies already carried out regarding symptom management within children's palliative care focus on children with cancer. Further research should continue to develop these, but also examine symptom management for children with other life-limiting illness, whether at the end of life or extended over many years.

This chapter has outlined the key symptoms that children frequently experience, and discussed the management of these symptoms from a practice perspective. The diversity of conditions, and therefore symptoms, that children experience can present challenges to those caring for them. Central to the assessment and management of children's symptoms is the need to work in partnership with both the child and the parents, and recognize them as experts in the child's care. As with the other aspects of care discussed in this book, symptom management must adopt an interdisciplinary approach (Beardsmore and Fitzmaurice 2002). Listening actively to children and their parents, and sharing expertise and knowledge within the health care team are key issues in symptom management from the time of the child's diagnosis until the end-of-life phase.

Key resources

Goldman, A., Hain, R. and Liben, S. (2006) *Oxford Textbook of Palliative Care for Children*. Oxford: Oxford University Press.

Jassal, S. (2008) *Basic Symptom Control in Paediatric Palliative Care: The Rainbows Hospice Guidelines*, 7th edn. Available at: www.act.org.uk

Paedpalcare mailing list. Available at: www.act.org.uk

CHAPTER SUMMARY

- The evidence-based underpinning symptom management in children requiring palliative care requires further development.

- Issues can arise, as many drugs used in adult symptom management are not licensed for use with children.

- The assessment and management of a child's symptoms is a continuous and ongoing process throughout the child's illness trajectory.

- Pain is one of the most common symptoms experienced by children with life-limiting conditions.

- Symptom management must include both the child and the family, and should include pharmacological and non-pharmacological interventions.

- Effective use of the interdisciplinary team makes symptom management more effective and efficient.

References

ACT and RCPCH (Association for Children with Life-threatening or Terminal Conditions and their Families and the Royal College of Paediatrics and Child Health) (2003) *A Guide to the Development of Children's Palliative Care Services Report of a Joint Working Party of the Association for Children with Life-Threatening or Terminal Conditions and their Families* (2nd edn) Bristol: ACT .

Anghelescu, D., Oakes, L., Hinds, P. (2006) Palliative care and pediatrics. *Anaesthesiology Clinic of North America* **24**: 145–61.

Asantila, R., Eklund, P. and Rosenberg, P. H., (1993) Epidural analgesia with 4 mg of morphine following caesarean section: effect of injected volume. *Acta Anaesthesiologica Scandinavica* **37**: 764–7.

Ashton, H. (1994) Guidelines for the rational use of benzodiazepines. When and what to use. *Drugs* **48**: 25–40.

Bais, J. E., Horbach, T. L., Masclee, A. A., Smout, A. J., Terpstra, J.L. and Gooszen, H. G. (2000) Surgical treatment for recurrent gastro-oesophageal reflux disease after failed antireflux surgery. *British Journal of Surgery* **87**: 243–9.

Beardsmore, S. and Fitzmaurice, N. (2002) Palliative care in paediatric oncology. *European Journal of Cancer* **38**: 1900–07; discussion, 1908–10.

Bellomo-Brandao, M. A., Collares, E. F. and da-Costa-Pinto, E. A. (2003) Use of erythromycin for the treatment of severe chronic constipation in children. *Brazilian Journal of Medical and Biological Research* **36**: 1391–6.

Blasco, P. A. and Stansbury, J. C. (1996) Glycopyrrolate treatment of chronic drooling. *Archives of Pediatrics and Adolescent Medicine* **150**: 932–5.

Blume, W. T. (1992) Uncontrolled epilepsy in children. *Epilepsy Res Suppl* **5**: 19–24.

Breau, L. M., Camfield, C., McGrath, P. J., Rosmus, C. and Finley, G. A. (2001) Measuring pain accurately in children with cognitive impairments: refinements of a caregiver scale. *Journal of Pediatrics* **138**(5): 721–7.

British National Formulary for Children (BNFC) (2008) London: British Medical Association, the Royal Pharmaceutical Society of Great Britain, the Royal College of Paediatrics and Child Health, and the Neonatal and Paediatric Pharmacists Group.

Brown, E. (2007) Managing children's pain. In Brown, E. with Warr, B. *Supporting the child and the family in paediatric palliative care.* London: Jessica Kingsley.

Burtles, R. and Astley, B. (1983) Lorazepam in children. A double-blind trial comparing lorazepam, diazepam, trimeprazine and placebo. *British Journal of Anaesthesia* **55**: 275–9.

Camfield, P. R. (1999) Buccal midazolam and rectal diazepam for treatment of prolonged seizures in childhood and adolescence: a randomised trial. *The Journal of Pediatrics* **135**: 398–9.

Candy, D.C., Edwards, D. and Geraint, M. (2006) Treatment of faecal impaction with polyethelene glycol plus electrolytes (PGE + E) followed by a double-blind comparison of PEG + E versus lactulose as maintenance therapy. *Journal of Pediatric Gastroenterology and Nutrition* **43**: 65–70.

Ceriati, E., De Peppo, F., Ciprandi, G., Marchetti, P., Silveri, M. and Rivosecchi, M. (2006) Surgery in disabled children: general gastroenterological aspects. *Acta Paediatrica (Supplement)* **95**: 34–7.

Choonara, I. (2004) Unlicensed and off-label drug use in children: implications for safety. *Expert Opinion on Drug Safety* **3**: 81–3.

Collins, J. J., Byrnes, M. E., Dunkel, I. J., Lapin, J., Nadel, T., Thaler, H. T., Polyak, T., Rapkin, B. and Portenoy, R. K. (2000) The measurement of symptoms in children with cancer. *Journal of Pain and Symptom Management* **19**: 363–77.

Collins, J. J. and Fitzgerald, D. A. (2006) Palliative care and paediatric respiratory medicine. *Paediatric Respiratory Reviews* **7**: 281–7.

Czarnecki, M. L., Jandrisevits, M. D., Theiler, S. C., Huth, M.M. and Weisman, S. J. (2004) Controlled-release oxycodone for the management of pediatric postoperative pain. *Journal of Pain and Symptom Management* **27**: 379–86.

Demol, P., Ruoff, H. J. and Weihrauch, T. R. (1989) Rational pharmacotherapy of gastrointestinal motility disorders. *European Journal of Pediatrics* **148**: 489–95.

Dowling, M. (2004) Pain assessment in children with neurological impairment. *Paediatric Nursing* **16**(3): 37–8.

Drake, R. and Hain, R. (2006) Pain – pharmacological management. In Goldman, A., Hain, R. and Liben, S. (eds) *Oxford Textbook of Palliative Care for Children.* Oxford: Oxford University Press.

Durant, P. A. and Yaksh, T. L. (1988) Drug effects on urinary bladder tone during spinal morphine-induced inhibition of the micturition reflex in unanesthetized rats. *Anesthesiology* **68**: 325–34.

Duval, M. and Wood, C. (2002) Treatment of non-painful symptoms in terminally ill children. *Archives of Pediatrics* **9**: 1173–8.

Dyregrov, K. (2004) Bereaved parents' experience of research participation. *Social Science & Medicine* **58**: 391–400.

Emery, E. (2003) Intrathecal baclofen. Literature review of the results and complications. *Neurochirurgie* **49**: 276–88.

Emslie, G. J., Kennard, B. D., Mayes, T. L., Nightingale-Teresi, J., Carmody, T., Hughes, C. W., Rush, A. J., Tao, R. and Rintelmann, J. W. (2008) Fluoxetine versus placebo in preventing relapse of major depression in children and adolescents. *American Jjournal of Psychiatry* **165**: 459–67.

Fogarasi, A., Janszky, J. and Tuxhorn, I. (2006) Autonomic symptoms during childhood partial epileptic seizures. *Epilepsia* **47**: 584–8.

Frager, G., Collins, J. J. (2006) *Oxford Textbook of Palliative Care for Children*. Oxford: Oxford University Press.

Friedrichsdorf, S. J. and Collins, J. J. (2007) Management of non-pain symptoms in pediatric palliative care. *Medical Principles and Practice* **16** (Supplement): 3–9.

Friedrichsdorf, S. J. and Kang, T. I. (2007) The management of pain in children with life-limiting illnesses. *The Pediatric Clinics of North America* **54**: 645–72.

Gold, B. D. (2004) Review article: epidemiology and management of gastro-oesophageal reflux in children. *Alimentary Pharmacology and Therapeutics* **19**(Supplement 1): 22–7.

Golden, A. S., Haut, S. R. and Moshe, S. L. (2006) Nonepileptic uses of antiepileptic drugs in children and adolescents. *Pediatric Neurology* **34**: 421–32.

Goldman, A. and Burne, R. (1998) Symptom management. In Goldman, A. (ed.) *Care of the Dying Child*. Oxford: Oxford University Press.

Goldman, A., Hewitt, M., Collins, G. S., Childs, M. and Hain, R. (2006) Symptoms of children/young people with progressive malignant disease: United Kingdom children's cancer study group/paediatric oncology nurses forum survey. *Pediatrics* **117**(6): e1179–e1186.

Graham, R. J. and Robinson, W. M. (2005) Integrating palliative care into chronic care for children with severe neurodevelopmental disabilities. *Journal of Developmental and Behavioural Pediatrics* **26**: 361–5.

Grimshaw, D., Holroyd, E., Anthony, D. and Hall, D. M. (1995) Subcutaneous midazolam, diamorphine and hyoscine infusion in palliative care of a child with neurodegenerative disease. *Child Care, Health and Development* **21**: 377–81.

Hain, R. and Wallace, A. (2008) Progress in palliative care for children. *Paediatrics and Child Health* **18**: 141–6.

Hetrick, S., Merry, S., McKenzie, J., Sindahl, P. and Proctor, M. (2007) Selective serotonin reuptake inhibitors (SSRIs) for depressive disorders in children and adolescents. *Cochrane Database of Systematic Reviews (online)*, CD004851.

Hewitt, M., Goldman, A., Collins, G. S., Childs, M. and Hain, R. (2008) Opioid use in palliative care of children and young people with cancer. *Journal of Pediatrics* **152**: 39–44.

Hinds, P. S., Fouladi, M., Furman, W. L., Spunt, S. L., Drew, D., Oakes, L. L. and Church, C. (2005) End-of-life care preferences of pediatric patients with cancer. *Journal of Clinical Oncology* **23**: 9146–54.

Hinds, P. S., Wolfe, J., Schum, L. and Baker, J.N. (2005) Key factors affecting dying children and their families. *Journal of Palliative Medicine* 8(Suppl1): S70–S78.

Houlahan, K. E., Dinning, C., McCabe, M., Branowicki, P. A. and Mack, J. W. (2006) Can end of life care for the pediatric patient suffering with escalating and intractable symptoms be improved? *Journal of Pediatric Oncology Nursing* **23**: 45–51.

Hunt, A., Goldman, A., Devine, T. and Phillips, M. (2001) Transdermal fentanyl for pain relief in a paediatric palliative care population. *Palliative Medicine* **15**: 405–12.

Hunt, A., Mastroyannopoulou, K., Goldman, A. and Seers, K. (2003) Not knowing – the problem of pain in children with severe neurological impairment. *International Journal of Nursing Studies* **40**: 171–83.

Jassal, S. (2008) *Basic Symptom Control in Paediatric Palliative Care: The Rainbows Hospice Guidelines,* 7th edn. Available at: www.act.org.uk

Keady, S. (2007) Update on drugs for gastro-oesophageal reflux disease. *Archives of Disease in Childhood – Education and Practice* **92**: 114–18.

Klepstad, P., Kaasa, S., Cherny, N., Hanks, G. and de Conno, F. (2005) Pain and pain treatments in European palliative care units. A cross sectional survey from the European Association for Palliative Care Research Network. *Palliative Medicine* **19**: 477–84.

Lago, P. M., Bergounioux, J., Piva, J. P. and Devictor, D. (2007) End-of-life care in children: the Brazilian and the international perspectives. *Journal de Pediatria* **83**: S109-S116.

Lavy, V. (2007) Presenting symptoms and signs in children referred for palliative care in Malawi. *Palliative Medicine* **21**: 333–9.

Lehwald, N., Krausch, M., Franke, C., Assmann, B., Adam, R. and Knoefel, W. T. (2007) Sandifer syndrome – a multidisciplinary diagnostic and therapeutic challenge. *European Journal of Pediatric Surgery* **17**: 203–6.

Li, S. T., Grossman, D. C. and Cummings, P. (2007) Loperamide therapy for acute diarrhea in children: systematic review and meta-analysis. *PLoS Medicine* (Public Library of Science) **4**: e98.

Massimo, L. (2001) Home care services and the role of 'caregivers'. *Minerva Pediatrica* **53**: 161–9.

Mathew. A., Mathew, M. C., Thomas, M. and Antonisamy, B. (2005) The efficacy of diazepam in enhancing motor function in children with spastic cerebral palsy. *Journal of Tropical Pediatrics* **51**: 109–13.

McCallum, D. E., Byrne, P. and Bruera, E. (2000) How children die in hospital. *Journal of Pain Symptom Management* **20**: 417–23.

McCluggage. H.-L. and Elborn, J. S. (2006) Symptoms suffered by life-limited children that cause anxiety to UK children's hospice staff. *International Journal of Palliative Nursing* **12**: 254–8.

McNeilly, P, Price, J. and McCloskey, S. (2004) The use of syringe drivers – a paediatric perspective. *International Journal of Palliative Nursing* **1**(8): 399–403.

Michelson, K. N. and Steinhorn, D. M. (2007) Pediatric end-of-life issues and palliative care. *Clinical Pediatric Emergency Medicine* **8**: 212–19.

Motta. F., Buonaguro. V. and Stignani. C. (2007) The use of intrathecal baclofen pump implants in children and adolescents: safety and complications in 200 consecutive cases. *Journal of Neurosurgery* **107**: 32–5.

Murphy, J. V., Dehkaharghani, F. (1994) Diagnosis of childhood seizure disorders. *Epilepsia* **35**(Suppl 2): S7-S17.

NICE (National Institute for Health and Clinical Excellence) (2004) Newer drugs for epilepsy in children. Available at: www.nice.org.uk

Noyes, M. and Irving, H. (2001) The use of transdermal fentanyl in pediatric oncology palliative care. *American Journal of Hospice and Palliative Medicine* **18**: 411–16.

O'Neill, J. and Fountain, A. (1999) Levomepromazine (methotrimeprazine) and the last 48 hours. *Hospital Medicine* **60**: 564–7.

Pashankar, D. S. and Bishop, W. P. (2001) Efficacy and optimal dose of daily polyethylene glycol 3350 for treatment of constipation and encopresis in children. *The Journal of Pediatrics*: 661–4.

Prasad, A. N., Stafstrom, C. F. and Holmes, G. L. (1996) Alternative epilepsy therapies: the ketogenic diet, immunoglobulins, and steroids. *Epilepsia* **37**(Suppl 1): S81-S95.

Prince's Foundation for Integrated Health, The (2007) *Complementary Healthcare: A Guide for Patients.* Available at: www.fih.org.uk/document.rm?id=19

Prince's Foundation for Integrated Health, The, and the National Council for Hospice and Specialist Palliative Care Services (2003) *National Guidelines for the Use of Complementary Therapies in*

Supportive and Palliative Care. Available at: www.fih.org.uk/information_library/publications/health_guidelines/complementary.html

Rushton, C. H., Comello, K., Sellers, D. E., Reder, E., Hall, B. and Hutton, N. (2006) Interdisciplinary interventions to improve pediatric palliative care and reduce health care professional suffering. *Journal of Palliative Medicine* **9**: 922–33.

Salvatore, S. and Vandenplas, Y. (2003) Gastro-oesophageal reflux disease and motility disorders. *Best Practice and Research in Clinical Gastroenterology* **17**: 163–79.

Salvatore, S., Hauser, B. and Vandenplas, Y. (2004) The natural course of gastro-oesophageal reflux. *Acta Paediatrica* **93**: 1063–9.

Santucci, G. and Mack, J. W. (2007) Common gastrointestinal symptoms in pediatric palliative care: nausea, vomiting, constipation, anorexia, cachexia. *The Pediatric Clinics of North America* **54**: 673–89.

Scott, R. C., Besag, F. M. and Neville, B. G. (1999) Buccal midazolam and rectal diazepam for treatment of prolonged seizures in childhood and adolescence: a randomised trial. *Lancet* **353**: 623–6.

Simonds, A. K. (2006) Recent advances in respiratory care for neuromuscular disease. *Chest* **130**: 1879–86.

Sourkes, B., Frankel, L., Brown, M., Contro, N., Benitz, W., Case, C., Good, J., Jones, L., Komejan, J, Modderman-Marshall, H., Reichard, W., Sentivany-Collins, S. and Sunde, C. (2005) Food, toys and love: pediatric palliative care. *Current Problems in Pediatric Adolescent Health Care*, **35**: 350–86.

Stirling, L C., Kurowska, A. and Tookman, A. (1999) The use of phenobarbitone in the management of agitation and seizures at the end of life. *Journal of Pain Symptom Management* **17**: 363–8.

Swerdlow, M. (1980) The treatment of 'shooting' pain. *Postgraduate Medical Journal* **56**: 159–61.

Theuissen, J. M. J., Hoogerbrugge, P. M., van Acterberg, T., Prins, J. B., Vernooij-Dassen, M. J. F. J. and van den Ende, C. H. M. (2007) Symptoms in the palliative phase of children with cancer. *Pediatric Blood Cancer*, **49**: 160–5.

Thomson, M. A., Jenkins, H. R., Bisset, W. M. , Heuschkel, R., Kalra, D. S., Green, M. R., Wilson, D. C. and Geraint, M. (2007) Polyethylene glycol 3350 plus electrolytes for chronic constipation in children: a double blind, placebo controlled, crossover study. *Archives of Disease in Childhood* **92**: 996–1000.

Tscheng, D. Z. (2002) Sialorrhea – therapeutic drug options. *Annals of Pharmacotherapy* **36**: 1785–90.

Twycross, A., Moriarty, A. and Betts, T. (1998) *Paediatric Pain Management: A Multidisciplinary Approach*. London: Radcliffe Medical Press.

Ullrich, C. K. and Mayer, O. H. (2007) Assessment and management of fatigue and dyspnea in pediatric palliative care. *The Pediatric Clinics of North America* **54**: 735–56.

Van der Burg, J. J., Jongerius, P.H., Van Hulst, K., Van Limbeek, J. and Rotteveel, J. J. (2006) Drooling in children with cerebral palsy: effect of salivary flow reduction on daily life and care. *Developmental Medicine and Child Neurology* **48**: 103–7.

Viola, R., Kiteley, C., Lloyd, N. S., Mackay, J. A., Wilson, J. and Wong, R. K. (2008) The management of dyspnea in cancer patients: a systematic review. *Support Care Cancer* **16**: 329–37.

Wallace, J. D. (1994) Summary of combined clinical analysis of controlled clinical trials with tizanidine. *Neurology* **44**: S60-S68; discussion, S68-S69.

Watterson, G. and Hain, R. D. W. (2003) Palliative care: moving forward. *Current Paediatrics* **13**: 221–5.

Whittam, E. H. (1993) Terminal care of the dying child: psychosocial implications of care. *Cancer* **71**: 3450–62.

Willis, E (2007) Symptom care flowcharts: a case study. *Paediatric Nursing* **19**(1): 14–17.

Wolfe, J., Grier, H. E., Klar, N., Levin, S. B., Ellenbogen, J. M., Salem-Schatz, S., Emanuel, E. J. and Weeks, J. C. (2000) Symptoms and suffering at the end of life in children with cancer. *New England Journal of Medicine* **342**: 326–33.

Wolfe, J., Hammel, J. F., Edwards, K. E., Duncan, J., Comeau, M., Breyer, J., Aldridge, S., Grier, H. E., Berde, C., Dussel, V., and Weeks, J. C. (2008) *Journal of Clinical Oncology* **26**: 1717–23.

Wong, D. and Baker, C. (1998) Pain in children: comparison of assessment scales in children. *Pediatric Nursing* **14**: 9–17.

Wong. I., Sweis, D., Cope, J. and Florence, A. (2003) Paediatric medicines research in the UK: how to move forward? *Drug Safety* **26**: 529–37.

World Health Organization (1998) *Cancer Pain Relief and Palliative Care in Children.* WHO.

Zhdanova, I. V. (2005) Melatonin as a hypnotic: pro. *Sleep Medicine Reviews* **9**: 51–65.

CHAPTER 9

Caring for the Child at the End of Life

Ruth Davies

Introduction

Despite all our best efforts, children and young people still die from life-limiting conditions. The aim of this chapter is to discuss current service provision in relation to their end-of-life care, and identify the best of evidence-based practice. The focus at this stage must be on meeting the needs and wishes of the dying child or young person and their family, and for this reason the chapter will show how the ACT (2004) Care Pathway can facilitate this in practice. Having lost a much-loved teenage son to cancer, I write with personal as well as professional conviction about the importance of a 'good death'; that is, one that is dignified and pain-free. I believe this is the goal of high-quality end-of-life care, and an achievable one, but only if professionals commit to this ideal and apply a systematic, evidence-based approach to care in practice. Meeting the needs and wishes of the dying child or young person as well as their family is essential if we are to achieve a 'good death'. This, in my estimation, is the alpha and omega of high-quality end-of-life care.

KEY POINT
Meeting the needs and wishes of the child and family is essential if high-quality end-of-life care is to be achieved.

History and policy context of end-of-life care

Less than a century ago, end-of-life care for the majority of children and young people in the developed world would have been at home. However, the rise of hospital medicine from the 1940s began the trend for most people, including children and young people, to die in hospital wards or specialized units for cancer or intensive care. However, from the 1980s, those working with dying children and their families were beginning to question this practice, with home care being advocated as one of the better alternatives. This new thinking was no doubt influenced by developments in adult and paediatric palliative care, and a philosophy that placed emphasis on individual choice, both in the manner and the place of death. However, despite a clear preference for end-of-life care at home by children and/or their families across many countries, including Australia (The National Palliative Care Program 2004), Canada (Widger et al. 2007), Greece (Papadatou et al. 1996), Ireland (Department of Health and Children 2005), Poland (Dangel 2002), the UK (Andrews and Hood 2003, Vickers et al. 2007) and the USA (Belasco et al. 2000), most continue to die in hospital.

Variation in the provision of community-based palliative care services across the developed world means that a home death may not be a reality for many children with life-limiting conditions or their families. Within the UK, a House of Commons Report (2004) acknowledged that whether children receive palliative care services is dependent on their condition as well as geography. Since the 1980s an increasing number of children with malignant life-limiting conditions (leukaemias and solid tumours, for example) have been able to die at home because there are paediatric outreach oncology nurses attached to regional paediatric oncology centres (Beardsmore and Fitzmaurice 2002; Vickers et al. 2007). However, children with non-malignant conditions, which represent the majority of life-limiting conditions, are less likely to have this option, because of a general lack of community-based paediatric -nursing teams with palliative expertise. This is evident from a small epidemiological study of mortality in children and young people aged 0–19 years in Cardiff, Wales (Davies 2003) which identified that, while a quarter of all deaths between 1990–5 were as a result of life-limiting conditions, less than a third died at home. This study identified that the majority of home deaths were those from cancer, supported by the paediatric outreach oncology nurses operating out of the local United Kingdom Children's Cancer Study Group (UKCCSG) centre; in comparison, no such community-based palliative care service was available for those with non-malignant life-limiting conditions.

Despite a general assumption that children and young people with malignant conditions such as leukaemia and solid tumours are more likely to have a choice and to die at home (Beardsmore and Fitzmaurice 2002), this is not always the case. Higginson and Thompson's (2003) study of death registrations for all cancer deaths in England between 1995 and 1999 for children, aged 0–15 years and young people aged 16–24 years, found that only 52 per cent of children and 30 per cent of young people died at home, and that being from a lower social class, living in Inner London or in an area of high childhood poverty reduced the likelihood of a home death. This is reflected in Feudtner et al.'s (2002) study of place of death for children aged 1–18 years in Washington state, USA, which found that while home deaths had risen from 21 per cent to 43 per cent between 1980 and 1998, children living in poorer neighbourhoods, regardless of their condition, were less likely to die at home. A range of factors militate against a home death, and these, as Feudtner *et al.* observe, may include social and cultural issues, the unpredictability of death for some conditions as well as patterns of suffering and symptoms; any of these can make the process of dying at home 'extraordinarily difficult, frightening or otherwise untenable' for families (2002: 5).

ACTIVITY

Consider the possible advantages for a family to have their child's end-of-life care delivered at home.

While home may be regarded as the most appropriate environment for care, this may not be possible, or even desirable, for some families. There may, as Dominica (1987) has observed, be unwillingness by parents to want to live in a home where their child has died, and even the desire by the dying child for their parents to be in a protective and supportive environment. Understandably, some parents may feel totally overwhelmed by caring for their dying child alongside other family and home responsibilities. This may be particularly difficult for single parents, who have to bear the care of their dying child alone and unsupported, or who, as in the case of James referred to below, have the added burden of poverty.

CLINICAL FOCUS

James, a 10-year-old boy suffered from Niemann Pick syndrome, a rare genetic neurodegenerative condition, lived with his single, unsupported mother, younger brother aged 7 years (who had the same life-limiting condition) and two younger sisters, aged 5 and 3 years of age. The family home was three small rooms in a condemned Victorian house situated in a deprived inner city area. James's father had had little contact with his family since a court order was served on him following physical abuse towards his wife and children. James's mother opted for her son to receive end-of-life care at the local children's hospice. Over the previous four years, James, his mother and siblings had enjoyed family respite and had built up close relationships with the hospice staff and family link worker. His mother noted:

'I wanted J to have dignity and I wanted to be with him as much as possible, and if he'd been at home there's no way I could've done what was done for him. I have so much praise for the way they cared for him.'

James's mother agreed on an end-of-life care plan with the hospice staff, who respected her wish for him not to be resuscitated. She felt he had a good death in that he was pain-free and that the staff were caring and kind towards not only him but also them as a family. At her request, his funeral service was held at the hospice, and staff helped her with the funeral arrangements, including registering his death. Since James's death, his brother continues to receive respite at the hospice while his sisters attend the sibling bereavement support group. The ongoing post-bereavement support his mother receives from the family link worker and hospice continues to be helpful to her. The mother said:

'I felt she was there to help me. I could talk to her. I felt she was there, even now. And that with the hospice, just because your child died doesn't mean "It's over you know, you've had our help." You can still go there. You still meet up and have "get-togethers", which I go to with parents. You keep in contact and I think that's something that is needed.'

Adapted excerpt from Davies (2002).

End-of-life care in a children's hospice may be the preferred option for both children and their families. They can provide what some homes and most acute hospital environments cannot, and that is quiet, unhurried care in a private and purpose-designed environment so that parents can spend as much of the precious remaining time that is left with their dying child as well as with their child's body after death (Gold 1997). This environment of care gives parents the time, space and privacy they need through the whole of the end-of-life care stage, and can be a source of comfort to them not only at the time of their child's death but also in their bereavement (Davies 2005).

Even so, children's hospices are not accessible to all dying children or their families. Funded by local charities, they have not been planned strategically and so are not available in some parts of the UK or in many developed countries. Within the UK there are now more than forty children's hospices, with more planned, while some have also been set up Australia, Canada and the USA. Some UK-based ones are able to offer end-of-life care at home, and it should be noted that this form of 'hospice at home' is available in parts of Poland as well as Belarus. Unfortunately, most only accept children up to the age of 18 or 19 years of age, so excludes the increasing number of young people with life-limiting conditions who are now surviving into their twenties and beyond. Some children's hospices in the UK also provide adolescent hospices, but these are the exception rather the rule (ACT 2007). In any case, few children die within these (Dominica 1987).

KEY POINT

End-of-life care for children may be delivered in hospital, at home or in a hospice.

End-of-life care for the majority of children and young people with life-limiting conditions in the developed world will take place in hospital, within general wards or specialized units for intensive care or cancer, and even in accident and emergency departments. Children and young people may even choose to die in hospital. Feudtner et al. (2002) note that some adolescents, after years of living with a life-limiting condition, prefer to be in this familiar environment, especially if the demands of care are overwhelming and there is a lack of community-based palliative services. However, it has to be acknowledged that hospitals are geared to acute, intensive and curative treatment rather than palliation, and may not necessarily meet the end-of-life care needs of the child or young person or their family because of a lack of expertise in palliative care (Liben et al. 2008).

=== **FURTHER READING** ===

Read Andrews, F. and Hood, P. (2003) Shared care: hospital, hospice, home. *Paediatric Nursing* **6**: 20–2. Consider how an integrated interdisciplinary team approach improved the care for the child and family.

End-of-life care pathways

Meeting in full the end-of-life care needs of the child or young person, as well as their family, should be the goal of any civilized society, and this should be provided in whatever setting they die. To achieve this, new ways of working need to be put in place because, as the WHO (2004) note, knowledge about effective care rarely leads to widespread improvement without a deliberate effort being

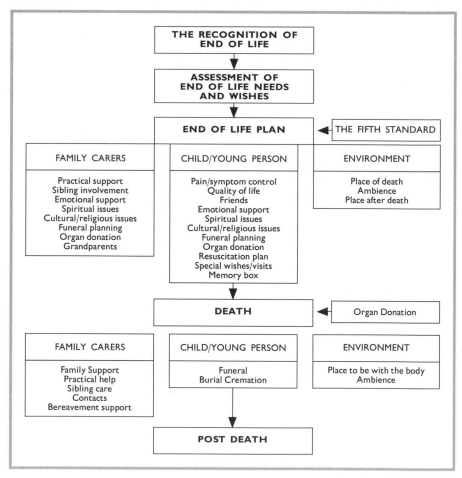

Figure 9.1 End-of-life care pathway

Source: ACT (2004). Reproduced with the kind permission of ACT.

made to change practice. In this respect, care pathways may provide the means of assessing, planning and implementing high-quality co-ordinated care at the end-of-life stage. To this end, the integrated multi-agency care pathway, developed by ACT (2004) with the Royal College of Nursing (RCN) and the Royal College of Paediatrics and Child Health (RCPCH), in conjunction with parents, social workers and educationalists, provides a systematic, evidence-based framework underpinned by a series of standards and key goals on which to base practice. Application of this pathway, shown in Figure 9.1, can, as will be seen later, provide the means of ensuring the end-of-life care needs and wishes of the dying child and their family are met effectively.

Recognition of end-of-life stage

Recognition of the end-of-life stage varies according to the life-limiting condition. It is not unknown for a child with severe cerebral palsy to deteriorate rapidly and die suddenly, whereas the same stage for a young man with muscular dystrophy may be protracted and take place over weeks rather than days. Similarly, for those with cancer, death may occur after periods of aggressive therapy. Families need to be treated with the utmost kindness when given this devastating news, as evidenced by Contro *et al.*'s (2002) study, which explored family perspectives on the quality of end-of-life care in a Californian children's hospital. Findings showed that parents preferred a familiar person to deliver this news, and stressed their need for this to be given with compassion and care using straightforward, non-technical language. Parents also valued honesty, clinical accuracy and open communication with caregivers. Early recognition and understanding of the prognosis by parents and practitioners can prevent needless suffering. Parents in studies by Wolfe, Grier *et al.* (2000) and Wolfe, Klar *et al.* (2000) reported that their child had experienced significant suffering and unrelieved pain in their last month of life when dying from advanced cancer. Their study also concluded that the integration of palliative care was considerably delayed because of unrealistic expectations on the part of physicians as well as parents, thus leading to inappropriate treatment. Accurate and honest prognosis, sooner rather than later, may avert such suffering, and end-of-life planning itself may help the child and family focus on quality of life rather than quantity.

Initial assessment of end-of-life care needs

The end-of-life care plan should be developed in partnership with the child or young person, wherever possible, and their family, and reflect individual needs rather than a formulaic plan of care. Shared documentation between agencies, including parent-held records, written in plain English, can allow not only a co-ordinated inter agency approach to care but an also effective use of resources during what can only be described as a harrowing time for the family. Ideally, planning should take place with the whole family, including siblings and grand-parents, giving them the opportunity to discuss their individual needs and wishes, and help to forestall a family crisis or breakdown in care. In assessing needs, professional carers must be sensitive to variations that exist in relation to cultural and spiritual values, as these have a direct impact on important aspects of paediatric palliative care. Liben *et al.* (2008) have helpfully drawn attention to the fact that some of the core principles of palliative care such as open disclosure and active participation by patients in decision-making, as well as open expression of feelings, developed initially in the USA and UK, may be unacceptable to families outside of tradition. They explain, for example, that in China it would be culturally inappropriate for a child to be involved in decision-making about care or treatment, and that even talking about the possibility of the child's death would be regarded as cursing them or hastening them to their end. It has to be acknowledged that these core principles are not universally applicable, being based on the Western ideal of a rights-based society. In accepting this, we can also accept that these may be applicable and even embraced by a majority of children and young people as well as their families in Western society. Suffice to say, the role of the professional carer is to determine preferences based on individual needs for all members of society, including those from ethnic or religious minorities.

Pain and symptom control

In Chapter 8, the importance of symptom control throughout the child's illness trajectory was discussed and here we re-iterate the importance of pain and symptom management, particularly at the end-of-life stage. The key to achieving this is a regular assessment of pain levels, and there are a range of pain tools available for this that are suitable for all stages of cognitive development. The WHO (1998) analgesic pain ladder, considered to be the gold standard of adult palliation, may be used effectively for those with both malignant and non-malignant life-limiting conditions, and in any care setting (Lidstone *et al.*, 2006; see also Chapter 8, Figure 8.4 in this volume). Successful management of pain requires 24-hour access to a paediatric palliative care specialist, paediatrician or specially trained GP and nurses, all of whom must be committed to ensuring that the child or young person is kept pain free. This cannot be stressed enough, because major research studies alert us to the fact that children and young people with cancer are continuing to suffer significant distress and unrelieved pain at the end of life (Wolfe, Grier *et al.* 2000, Kreicbergs 2005) in some acute hospital settings. Unrelieved pain at this stage is unpardonable, precisely because modern medicine does have the technical means to reduce nearly all pain. Failure to do so, as Solomon and Browning rightly point out, may be regarded as a 'symptom of insufficient commitment' (2005: 9055) rather than a technical failing. In this connection, more education and training of those responsible for pain and symptom control is necessary at all levels of medical and nursing practice (Liben *et al.* 2008) if children and young people are to achieve what many, including myself, subscribe to: their fundamental right to a dignified and pain-free death.

Other symptoms, including pain at the end-of-life stage, vary according to the life-limiting condition. A nationwide survey of symptoms in Swedish children with cancer during their last month of life, carried out by Jalmsell *et al.* (2006)

and based on parental reports, revealed an extensive range of these, the most frequently reported being physical fatigue, reduced mobility, pain and decreased appetite. This study highlighted that those with leukaemias and lymphomas suffered more frequently from pain, poor appetite and troublesome swellings/oedema. In comparison, those with brain tumours suffered more frequently from difficulties in swallowing, paralysis, reduced mobility, impaired speech and constipation. Parents of children aged 9–15 years reported a greater range of symptoms, but this may be because their child was sufficiently mature to describe and communicate them. A large-scale survey of twenty-two UKCCSG centres (Goldman *et al.* 2006) also found an extensive range of symptoms in children at the end-of-life stage. Data from this study identified that while pain can now be treated effectively, with access to skilled symptom control, others such as weakness, anorexia and problems with mobility, as well as neurological deficits, often remain intractable. As Wolfe *et al.*'s study (2000) indicates, children and young people suffer not only from physical pain but also psychological pain, including 'no fun' towards the end of life, which may well include depression and anxiety (Pao *et al.* 2006). For those with non-malignant life-limiting conditions, there are a range of symptoms that need amelioration, such as dyspnoea, constipation, nausea and fitting. In the final days or hours of life, the child or young person may be affected by the 'death rattle' or noisy breathing caused by excessive respiratory secretions, and this can be distressing to their family. As noted in Chapter 8, this can be dealt with effectively by the use of anti-cholinergic medication. Most symptoms are amenable to palliation, and careful forward planning using the end-of-life care plan should result in these being anticipated and dealt with as they occur. However, for those with intractable pain, palliative sedation may be the only option for a pain-free and dignified death (Solomon and Browning 2005).

Decision-making: including the child or young person and their family

Professional carers need to ensure that the child or young person, as well as family members, feel supported by them at this time. This means taking time to listen to their fears and worries and, if asked, offering gentle suggestions and ideas that may inform their decision-making. No life experience will have prepared the child/young person and family for what is a frightening experience, and understandably they may turn to professional carers for advice and guidance. Openness and truthfulness about all aspects of decision-making is helpful for all involved, including the professional themselves, and is respectful of the child or young person's autonomy. It has been shown that children as young as 10 years of age are able to understand the consequences of their actions and make end-of-life decisions with regard to resuscitation orders or whether to forego life- sustaining therapies in favour of palliative care (Hinds *et al.* 2005). Actively involving children who are cognitively competent as well as young people not only respects their autonomy but also gives them some sense of control over what remains of their life, and professional carers need to be to be mindful of this with regard to decision-making about continuation or withdrawal of treatment. This may relate to resuscitation orders, whether second-line chemotherapy should be started once standard therapy has failed, or whether overnight ventilation should continue for a young man at the end stage of muscular dystrophy. Ethical dilemmas, such as these, should be guided by the fundamental principle of palliative care, which is that interventions should only be offered if their potential benefits outweigh the burdens to patients (RCPCH 2004) (discussed in Chapter 5). However, discussion about profound issues such as these does not always take place, as evidenced by De Graves and Aranda's (2002) Australian study, which investigated the shift from cure to palliation through researching the medical records of eighteen children who died from cancer. Sadly, while physical aspects of care were well documented, there was little evidence of human-to-human aspects of care or processes of decision-making.

<hr>

ACTIVITY

Reflect on a child and family you were caring for when a complex end-of-life decision had to be made. Use a reflective model – for example, McNeilly, P., Price, J. and McCloskey, S. (2006) Reflection in children's palliative care: a model. *European Journal of Palliative Care* 13(1): 31–4 to guide your thinking. What did you learn from this situation, and how would this change your practice in the future?

<hr>

Involving the child or young person in end-of-life planning, including decision-making, means having to talk to them about their own impending death, which some parents and health professionals are not always able to do. As one Canadian study, by McCallum *et al.* (2000) found, these decisions are often deferred until very close to the time of death, and children and young people are rarely told they are dying. In this study, involving seventy-seven cases, only one child, a teenager, was told explicitly that he was dying, and it was noted that as result he was able to participate in his own care and dying. As one large-scale American study found (Contro *et al.* 2002), the majority of health care professionals, including doctors, find themselves unable to discuss issues such as resuscitation or pain management with children or their parents. Involving parents may be seen as crucial in achieving the best outcome for the child or young person, as they play a major role in any decision-making process, with or without their child's input. Taking account of what is supportive to them is essential as shown by Meyer *et al.*'s (2006) study into improving quality of end-of-life care in three paediatric intensive care units in Boston, USA. This extensive study involved more than fifty parents whose child had died after withdrawal of life support, and resulted in them identifying six priorities for care. These were: honest and complete communication with care givers; ready access to staff; care co-ordination; emotional expression and support by staff; preservation of the parent–child relationship; and faith. All of these studies show, at a very human level, the need for everyone involved to be in open and honest communication with each other concerning end-of-life decision-making. End-of-life care planning must take this into account, with decisions documented on the actual plan to prevent any distressing and unnecessary interventions later. Enabling the family to talk openly about these sensitive issues may lead to open discussion and decisions about other aspects, such as organ donation and post mortem, which may also be helpful to the family and again guard against any misunderstandings or distress later on.

Quality of life at the end stage

Quality of life is an elusive concept, and how health care professionals through their caring practices can best support families to achieve this is probably best summed up by Sister Frances Dominica, who, in describing hospice care, writes; 'care is about being alongside those whose lifespan is short helping them to live until they die; it is about seeing time in terms of depth rather than length' (1987: 343). Quality of life to the child and young person will probably mean being surrounded by the love of family and friends, and making the most of any remaining time with pleasurable activities. This may involve seeing and being with friends, attending a party or a pop concert, watching favourite television programmes or videos, or listening to music. Supporting the child or young person to do what is important and pleasurable to them should be the goal, and these activities may well create a source of positive memories for the loved ones they leave behind.

Earlier chapters of this book have discussed the difficulties experienced by parents and professionals broaching the subject of death with their dying child. However, most of us who have cared for dying children and their families realize that even young children are aware in their own way that death is possible but, taking their cue from adults, do not talk about this to avoid causing them distress. Children may express their fears and anxieties about death in forms other than words, including via play or drawings (Bertoia 1993). Understanding how children themselves understand death may be helpful in meeting their end-of-life needs and wishes (this was discussed in Chapters 3 and 4). Useful as such understanding might be, it does not take into account that many children and young people with life-limiting conditions may already have experienced the loss of a fellow sufferer and therefore have an understanding beyond their years. In Faulkner's opinion, the goal of communicating with the dying child, in whatever form that takes, is to meet their particular needs, and this may be about 'correcting misconceptions, allaying fears, and reducing the isolation will make the transition from life to death easier for the child' (2001: 20).

KEY POINT

Regardless of the location of the child's end-of-life care, the family must remain at the centre of care and be involved in any decision-making.

Spiritual, religious and cultural issues at the end of life

The spiritual needs of children requiring palliative care, and their families, at the different stages of their illness trajectory have been discussed in Chapter 5.

Children and young people, no less than adults, have spiritual needs and, furthermore, fears and anxieties about dying. Thayer (2001) observes that a child or young person may have fears and anxieties about death, and about what will happen to them when they die. He posits that when they speak of heaven or the afterlife, their primary concern is 'Who will take care of me?' He reasons that to them this may be God or a relative who has already died, noting that their representations of heaven are usually concrete presentations of places where they are cared for in the same way as their parents care for them. Again, children no less than adults want to know that their life has made a difference and they are leaving an enduring legacy. Thayer suggests videotapes, sculptures and homemade books as ways of capturing the child's spirit. In this connection, memory boxes may also provide an enduring legacy, and some children and young people derive comfort from leaving gifts and possessions to family and friends.

Hospital chaplains, as well as priests and ministers affiliated to hospices and palliative care teams, are well versed in meeting the spiritual needs of the dying child or young person and their family. One study of hospital chaplains working in 115 children's hospitals across the USA (Feudtner et al. 2003) found that nearly a quarter of the children they were asked to visit were in fact dying. Chaplains in this study gave examples of spiritual distress they encountered in children as well as in their parents. For the child this included feeling fearful or anxious, coping with pain and other physical symptoms as well as relationships with their parents, or relationships between their parents. For parents, spiritual distress included questioning why they and their child were going through this experience, and about the meaning or purpose of suffering. Parents also expressed feelings of guilt because they could not prevent their child experiencing suffering or dying. Chaplains described some of the barriers they encountered in providing this care, cited inadequate training of health carers to detect spiritual distress, and of being invited to visit children and families too late to supply all the care that could have been provided.

For the parents of dying children, studies show that many acknowledge spirituality as being central to their efforts to draw some meaning from their child dying, as well providing guidance and permission around end-of-life decision-making (Feudtner 2003, Meyer et al. 2006). Gatrad et al. (2003) identified that some families from ethnic minorities in the UK have difficulty in accessing palliative care. Reasons include, the mistaken belief that some hospices, rooted in the Christian tradition, only cater for Christian communities, or that hospitals have 'unreasonable' restrictions on visiting times and the numbers of visitors allowed for dying patients. Issues such as these underline not only the need for unrestricted visiting, but also the importance of spiritual support as a key goal within of the end-of-life care pathway. To achieve this, we must ask the child and family what their needs and wishes are, document these, and ensure that they are met in full. Being open and receptive to the spiritual needs as well as religious beliefs and observances of all faiths in our multi-ethnic and multi-religious societies is essential if we are to provide a holistic approach to care.

Time of death: achieving a 'good death' for a child or young person and their family

Ellershaw and Ward (2003) identify from their work, based on many years of practice in adult palliative care as well as research inquiry, that a 'good death' is one that is pain-free and dignified, and in which active resuscitation does not take place. Ideally a 'good death' for the child or young person is also one that is pain free and dignified, in the environment of their choice and with those they love around them. Ensuring a 'good death' must be the goal, not only for the sake of the dying child/young person, but also for the sake of those who are left behind. Family and friends need to know and feel that a much loved child has experienced a 'good death', and this can be a source of comfort to them in their bereavement. Conversely, if the child or young person has experienced unresolved pain or symptom control during the end-of-life stage, this will be a source of anguish, especially to parents, for many years and probably for ever. Kreicbergs *et al.*'s (2005) nationwide study of Swedish parents whose child had died from cancer found that more than half reported that their child's pain could not be relieved and they were still deeply affected by this stressful experience between four and nine years after bereavement. Surkan *et al.* (2006) found that parents' perceptions of inadequate health care were also associated with feelings of guilt in the year following their child's death.

=== **ACTIVITY** ===

- What is a 'good death' for the child or young person?

- What is a 'good death' from a parent's perspective?

- Can you reflect on your own experience of a 'good' or a 'bad' death?

- What distinguishes these from each other in relation to aspects of care?

As noted earlier, death for some children and young people will take place in hospital, on wards, in intensive care units, in oncology centres or, if they deteriorate rapidly, in accident and emergency departments. Worryingly, as studies from different countries show, a hospital environment does not always provide what families need. Parents' accounts paint a bleak picture and show a lack of privacy for the dying child, and for them, in overcrowded, noisy and often poorly furnished and equipped hospital areas where the focus is on acute medical care rather than palliation (Papadatou *et al.* 1996, Steele 2002, Davies 2005). In this respect, it cannot be overstated that the dying child and his/her family need a room to themselves, giving them space, privacy and calmness. Regardless of which area of the hospital the child is in, parents, especially mothers, will want to continue as their child's main carer. As Meyer *et al.* (2006) have observed, professional carers are at their most helpful to parents when they honour the parents' rightful place at the centre of care, and make every effort to preserve the parent-child relationship. As they note, 'the continued presence and nurture of parents at the end of life has the potential to create dear and sustaining memories that begin to support the grieving process' (Meyer *et al.* 2006: 654).

Parents are the experts in their child's care and most have expert knowledge about their child's life-limiting condition. However, in today's society, few are acquainted with the reality of death, so they may need gentle preparation from health professionals about the physical changes that may occur in their child, such as increasing weakness, drowsiness or changes in skin colour. Pain and symptom control must be exemplary, and again, if the child is dying at home, parents should have enough analgesia so that dosage may be increased as and when required. This will be an exhausting time for all the family, but especially for the parents, who might appreciate help with their child's physical needs or, if they are at home, a night-sitting service. If at home, parents also need to be confident that help is at the end of a telephone, and that they have access to a 24-hour palliative care service that is both prompt and reliable. Identifying all these measures through forward planning and use of an end-of-life care plan may prevent family crisis or a breakdown in care that results in the child's admission to hospital.

This will be an extremely stressful time for other family members and friends, as well as the parents, and they may appreciate the use of a 'quiet room' where they can take some 'time out' and have the privacy to cry. Realistically, however, such a facility is rarely available in a busy NHS hospital and it may be that the only quiet space to be found will be in the hospital chapel. Whether the child is dying in hospital, at home or in a children's hospice, parents will want to carry on with their normal loving and caring practices, such as cuddling or talking to their child. Family and friends need to know that hearing is the last sense to go and, just because the child is unable to respond or is unconscious, it does not mean they cannot hear. Parents may therefore want to play their child's favourite music to them, or put on their favourite TV programme or video. Siblings, grandparents and other family members and friends may also want to spend time with the dying child, or just simply visit to say goodbye. At this stage, the child or young person and their family may need the solace and comfort of religious observances such as, baptism or the 'last rites' or other traditions such as family prayers. Once their child's life draws to its close, parents will probably want these very final and precious moments alone with them, and this should be respected. The role of the professional at this time is to help and support the needs and wishes of the child and their family. Use of the ACT (2004) care pathway can help to set out the goals that provide high-quality end-of-life care (RCN, 2004), as shown in the case of David, set out below.

After death

=========================== **ACTIVITY** ===========================

Read McNeilly, P. and Price, J. (2008) Care of the child after death, Chapter 44 in Kelsey, J. and McEwing, G. (eds), *Clinical Skills in Child Health Practice*. Oxford: Elsevier, and carefully consider carefully the care outlined after a child's death.

CLINICAL FOCUS
David: end-of-life care at home

David, aged 15 years, had advanced metastatic Ewing's sarcoma and wanted to die at home with his mother and younger sister.

Key goals in planning for end-of-life care (ACT, 2004)	Application in practice
Professionals should be open and honest with families when the approach of the end of life is recognized.	Clinical nurse specialist (CNS) visited mother and family as soon as possible. They wanted to know what would happen to David. CNS listened, answered questions, offered options and gave information about services.
Joint planning with families and relevant professionals should take place as soon as possible.	CNS identified as key worker Met with primary health care team (PHCT) and pain control team. Liaised and worked with GP. Spent time with siblings. Visited school at mother's request to support siblings.
A written plan of care should be agreed, including decisions about methods of resuscitation; emergency services should be informed.	Resuscitation plan agreed. Ambulance services informed.
Care plans should be reviewed and altered to take into account any changes.	Detailed care plan reviewed in response to changes in David's condition.
There should be 24-hour access to pain and symptom control, including access to medication.	David and family had access to 24/7 palliative care End-of-life care plan included pain and symptom control guidelines in medical and nursing documentation. Syringe pump provided and diamorphine and Nozinan titrated to take into account breakthrough pain. Medication available in family home. Safety measures put in place.
Those managing the control of symptoms should be suitably qualified and experienced.	Specialist lymphoedema nurse consulted about lymphoedema of left leg and scrotum. Pain control team, GP and PHCT worked closely with CNS.
Emotional and spiritual support should be available to the child and carers.	CNS spent time with David and family. CNS with David and family when he died, at their request.
Children and families should be supported in their choices and goals for quality of life to the end.	David visited by extended family and friends. Once he became paraplegic his mother and sister slept in same room with him, as he requested.

Following the death of a child or young person, the parents need to feel they can have privacy, quiet and time with their child's body. For some of these children, a post mortem may be required – if, for example, a definite diagnosis has not been reached. Parents need support and information regarding this, as it can be a cause of worry, anxiety and distress to the bereaved family (McNeilly and Price 2008).

=== **WEB LINKS** ===

Information for parents about post mortems is available at: www.dh.gov.uk/en/Publicationsandstatistics/Publications/PublicationsPolicyAndGuidance/DH_4130676

Parents should feel able to hold and cuddle their child, and to retain some sense of control over the child's body (ACT 2004). Their wishes at this stage need to be sought, especially with regard to whether they want to be involved in the laying out of their child. Health professionals need to be aware of any religious or cultural aspects of care, and it is hoped that these will have already been documented in the end-of-life care plan. Parents may want their child dressed in clothes that are meaningful to him/her or themselves, such as a football strip or bridesmaid's dress. They may also wish to take a lock of their child's hair, photographs, or in the case of a baby or small child, hand or footprints. Health professionals can best help parents at this time by letting them carry out their final acts of care in their own way (Dominica 1997). Parents should also feel that other siblings, family and friends can see their child's body if they wish to say final goodbyes. Providing fresh flowers in the child's room, religious symbols or other articles such as family photographs that are meaningful to them as a family is also helpful, and can ensure that their memories of this time are coloured by acts of kindness and reverence towards their child.

KEY POINT

Following the child's death, parents need time to be with their child and must be involved in care and choices at this time.

The family's wishes regarding where they want their child's body to be cared for should already be documented in the end-of-life care plan. If the child has died in hospital, parents may choose that they are transferred to the hospital mortuary and then on to a funeral director of their choice. Parents should always be asked if they wish to accompany their child's body to the hospital mortuary, and in my experience hospital porters and mortuary technicians are kind and supportive of this practice. Health professionals need to be informed about the legalities of practice. In the UK, for example, parents are entitled to take their child's body home if they wish, but as Whittle and Cutt's (2002) study found, they are not always informed of this option. If the child dies at home, parents may wish for their body to remain there, but will need advice and support from a funeral director. The role of the funeral director is outlined on p. 187.

CLINICAL FOCUS

Benjamin (Ben) a 9-year-old boy, who had previously been treated for leukaemia, died at home. His end-of-life care had been delivered there by his parents, his older sister and the interdisciplinary team.

Following Ben's death, his father contacted their GP, who visited their home and 'certified the death'. He then issued the Medical Certificate of Cause of Death often referred to as the Death Certificate. This certificate is needed in order to register the death.

Ben's father then contacted the local funeral director, who had been recommended by a family friend.

The Funeral Director arranged to visit the family at their own home to assist with the funeral arrangements. There he outlined the various options open to Ben's parents regarding the funeral service, type of coffin, transport, hymn sheets, funeral notices for the newspaper and so on.

They discussed the care and preparation of Ben's body, and his parents stated they wanted Ben dressed in his Manchester United football strip. The family decided they wanted Ben to return home to spend the two nights before his funeral in his bedroom. The parents made arrangements to move the furniture to facilitate the coffin and Ben's mother showed the funeral director the room and the space available.

The funeral director and the family discussed floral tributes and identified that they wanted any donations in lieu of flowers to go the local children's cancer ward.

INTERDISCIPLINARY INSIGHT

The role of the funeral director

- The Funeral Director will offer as much support as possible to Ben's family. He/she will explain fully what the procedure is at all points in the care of their son's body and planning for his funeral.

- The Funeral Director will be there for the family before, during and after the funeral, to assist with advice, care and guidance, or perhaps just a friendly chat.

- The Funeral Director discusses with and gives the parents options regarding the type of service, coffin and funeral for their son.

- To prepare and care for Ben's body.

- Give parents, siblings or others the opportunity to place toys, keepsakes and so on in Ben's coffin.

- Some Funeral Directors offer a Token of Remembrance Book, to enable family and friends to record their attendance at the funeral.

- Many Funeral Directors can help the family with supplying a new memorial stone or by adding wording to an existing memorial.

Written by Peter C. Mulholland, Funeral Home Manager

Parents whose child has died at a children's hospice may wish for them to remain in the 'special bedroom' (a room where the temperature may be lowered) so that family and friends can spend time with them in the days leading up to the funeral. For this reason, some parents whose child has received respite care at a children's hospice but has died at home or in hospital may ask for their child's body to transferred to the hospice (Davies 2005). The role of the professional at the time of death is to help and support the family to care for their child's body in the family's own way.

Conclusion

This chapter began with a discussion about place of death for the child or young person and whether this should be within hospital, at home or in a hospice. This highlighted the fact that, despite a preference by the majority to die in their own home, only a minority achieve this because of the lack of community-based palliative care services and expertise. Given that the majority of children and young people with life-limiting conditions will continue to die in hospital for the foreseeable future, there is an urgent need to integrate high-quality end-of-life care into all areas of hospital practice, while at the same time increasing community-based paediatric palliative care provision. It is a truism that those involved in the care of a dying child and his or her family have only one chance to get it right. This chapter has shown this is possible if we meet their needs and wishes and that a 'good death' is a realizable goal. It is also clear that high-quality end-of-life care does not just happen but is based on a systematic approach to evidence-based care (ACT 2004) which takes on board the need to work closely with individual families and members of the interdisciplinary team. I began this chapter by stating that, despite our best efforts, children and young people will continue to die from life-limiting conditions. We cannot prevent these deaths, but we can with sufficient commitment fulfill the ideal of a 'good death' and in doing so respect the fundamental right of every child or young person to die pain-free and with dignity.

Key resources

ACT (Association for Children with Life-threatening or Terminal Conditions and their Families) (2004) *A Framework for the Development of Integrated Multi-agency Care Pathways for Children with Life-threatening and Life-limiting Conditions*. Bristol, ACT.

Davies, R. (2005) Mothers' stories of loss: their need to be with their dying child and their child's body after death. *Journal of Child Health Care* 9(4): 288–300.

Lidstone, V., Delaney, J., Hain, R. and Jassal, S. S. (2006) *Paediatric Palliative Care Guidelines*, 2nd edn. South West London, Surrey, West Sussex and Hampshire, and Sussex Cancer Networks.

CHAPTER SUMMARY

- High quality end-of-life care focuses on meeting the needs and wishes of the child or young person and their family and is underpinned by the best evidence based practice.

- Ideally, the child or young person should have choice regarding place of death, this may include home, hospice or hospital.

- The ACT Integrated Multi-agency Care Pathway provides a systematic evidence based framework to assess, plan and implement high quality end-of-life care.

- Pain and symptom control must be exemplary and is possible if professionals are committed to the ideal of a child or young person's right to a 'good death'.

- Through the end-of-life care stage professionals must ensure that parents have their rightful place at the centre of care.

- After the child or young person's death, professionals must ensure that parents have privacy and time with their child's body.
- High quality end-of-life care is dependant upon professionals working closely with individual families and members of the interdisciplinary team.

Acknowledgement

My thanks to Brother Francis Worth for his contribution from practice.

References

ACT (Association for Children with Life-Threatening or Terminal Conditions and their Families) (2004) *A Framework for the Development of Integrated Multi-agency Care Pathways for Children with Life-threatening and Life-limiting Conditions*. Bristol: ACT.

ACT (Association for Children's Palliative Care) (2007) *The Transition Care Pathway: A Framework for the Development of Integrated Multi-agency Care Pathways for Children with Life-threatening and Life-limiting Conditions*. Bristol: ACT.

Andrews, F. and Hood, P. (2003) Shared care: hospital, hospice, home. *Paediatric Nursing* **6**: 20–2.

Beardsmore, S. and Fitzmaurice, N. (2002) Palliative care in paediatric oncology. *European Journal of Cancer* **38**(14): 1900–7.

Belasco, J. B., Danz, P., Drill, A., Schmid, W. and Burkey, E. (2000) Supportive care: palliative care in children, adolescents, and young adults – model of care, interventions, and cost of care: a retrospective review. *Journal of Palliative Care* **16**(4): 39–46.

Bertoia, J. (1993) *Drawings from a Dying Child*. London: Routledge.

Contro, N., Larson, J., Scofield, S., and Cohen, H. (2002) Family perspectives on quality of pediatric palliative care. *Archives of Pediatric and Adolescent Medicine* **156**: 14–19.

Dangel, T. (2002) The status of pediatric palliative care in Europe. *Journal of Pain and Symptom Management* **24**(2): 160–5.

Davies, R. (2002) A study of palliative care options for children and young people. Unpublished PhD thesis, University of Wales, College of Medicine.

Davies, R. (2003) Establishing need for palliative care services for children/young people. *British Journal of Nursing* **12**(4): 224–32.

Davies, R. (2005) Mothers' stories of loss: their need to be with their dying child and their child's body after death. *Journal of Child Health Care* **9**(4): 288–300.

De Graves, S. D. and Aranda, S. (2002) Exploring documentation of end-of-life care of children with cancer. *International Journal of Palliative Nursing* **8**(9): 435–43.

Department of Health and Children (2005) *Report on a Research Study of the Palliative Care Needs of Children in Ireland: Funded by the Department of Health and Children and the Irish Hospice.* Dublin: Stationery Office.

Dominica, F. (1987) The role of the hospice for the dying child. *British Journal of Hospital Medicine* October: 334–43.

Dominica, F. (1997) *Just My Reflection: Helping Parents to Do Things Their Way when Their Child Dies.* London: Darton, Longman and Todd.

Ellershaw, J., Ward, C. and Neuberger, J. (2003) Care of the dying patients: the last hours or days of life. *British Medical Journal* **326**: 30–4.

Faulkner, K. W. (2001) Children's understanding of death. In Armstrong-Dailey, A. and Zarbok, S. *Hospice Care for Children*, 2nd edn. Oxford: Oxford University Press.

Feudtner, C., Silveria, M. J. and Christakis, D. A. (2002) Where do children with complex chronic conditions die? Patterns in Washington state, 1980–1998. *Pediatrics* **109**(4): 656–60.

Feudtner, C., Haney, J. and Dimmers, M. A. (2003) Spiritual care needs of hospitalized children and their families: a national survey of pastoral care providers' perceptions. *Pediatrics* **111**(1): 67–72.

Gatrad, A. R., Brown, E. and Sheikh, A. (2003) Editorial: palliative care needs of minorities. *British Medical Journal* **327**: 176–7.

Gold, E. (1997) The role and need of the children's hospice in the United Kingdom. *International Journal of Palliative Nursing* **39**(5): 281–6.

Goldman, A., Hewitt, M., Collins, G. S., Childs, M. and Hain, R. (2006) Symptoms in children/young people with progressive malignant disease: United Kingdom Children's Cancer Study Group/Paediatric Oncology Nurses Forum Survey. *Pediatrics* **117**(6): 1179–86.

Higginson, I. J. and Thompson, M. (2003) Children and young people who die form from cancer: epidemiology and place of death in England. *British Medical Journal* **327**: 278–9.

Hinds, P. S., Drew, D., Oakes, L., Fouldadi, M., Spunt, S. L., Church, C. and Furman, W. L. (2005) End-of-life care preferences of pediatric patients with cancer. *Journal of Clinical Oncology* **23**: 9146–54.

House of Commons (2004) *Palliative Care: Fourth Report of Session 2003–04.* London: The Stationery Office.

Jalmsell, L., Kreicbergs, U., Onelov, E., Steineck, G. and Henter, J. (2006) Symptoms affecting children with malignancies during the last month of life: a nationwide follow-up *Pediatrics* **117**(4): 1314–20.

Kreicbergs, A., Validimarsdottir, U., Onelov, E., Bjork, O., Steineck, G., and Henter, J. (2005) Care-related distress: a nationwide study of parents who lost their child to cancer *Journal of Clinical Oncology* **23**(36): 9162–71.

Liben, S., Papadatou, D. and Wolfe, J. (2008) Paediatric palliative care: challenge and emerging ideas. *The Lancet.* Available at: www.the lancet.com/journals/lancet/articl/11SO1407612033; accessed 17 August 2008.

Lidstone, V., Delaney, J., Hain, R. and Jassal, S. S. (2006) *Paediatric Palliative Care Guidelines,* 2nd edn. South West London, Surrey, West Sussex and Hampshire, and Sussex Cancer Networks.

McCallum, D. E., Byrne, P. and Bruera, E. (2000) How children die in hospital. *Journal of Pain and Symptom Management* **20**(6): 417–23.

McNeilly , P. and Price, J. (2008) Care of the child after death. In Kelsey, J. and McEwing, G. (eds) Care of the child after death. *Clinical Skills in Child Health Practice.* Oxford: Elsevier.

McNeilly, P., Price, J. and McCloskey, S. (2006) Reflection in children's palliative care: a model. *European Journal of Palliative Care* **13**(1): 31–4.

Meyer, E. C., Ritholz, M. D., Burns, J. P. and Truog, R. D. (2006) Improving the quality of end-of-life care in the pediatric intensive care unit: parents' priorities and recommendations. *Pediatrics* **117**(3): 649–57.

National Palliative Care Program, The (2004) *Paediatric Palliative Care Service Model Review*. Canberra: Department of Health and Aging.

Pao, M., Balllard, E. D., Rosenstein, D. L., Wiener, L. and Wayne, A. S. (2006) Psychotropic medication use in pediatric patients with cancer. *Archives of Pediatrics and Adolescent Medicine* **160**(8): 818–22.

Papadatou, D., Yfantopoulos, J. and Kosmidis, H. V. (1996) Death of a child at home or in hospital: experiences of Greek mothers. *Death Studies* **20**: 215–35.

RCN (Royal College of Nursing) Abstract: Ruth Davies and Brother Francis Worth, *The development of the ACT palliative care pathway for children and young people*, Conference for Nurses Working with Children and Young People: York Racecourse, 1 October 2004.

RCPCH (Royal College of Paediatrics and Child Health) (2004) *Withholding or Withdrawing Life-Sustaining Treatment in Children: A Framework for Practice*, 2nd edn. London:, Royal College of Paediatrics and Child Health.

Solomon, M. Z. and Browning, D. (2005) Pediatric palliative care: relationships matter and so does pain control. *Journal of Clinical Oncology* **23**(36): 9055–7.

Steele, R. G. (2002) Experiences of families in which a child has a prolonged terminal illness: modifying factors. *International Journal of Palliative Nursing* **8**(9): 418–33.

Surkan, P. J., Kreicbergs, U., Valdimarsdottir, U., Nyberg, U., Onelov, E., Dickman, P. W. and Steineck, G. (2006) Perceptions of inadequate health care and feelings of guilt in parents after the death of a child to a malignancy: a population-based long-term follow-up. *Journal of Palliative Medicine* **9**(2): 317–31.

Thayer, P. (2001) Spiritual care of children and parents. In Armstrong-Dailey, A. and Zarbok, S. *Hospice Care for Children*, 2nd edn. Oxford: Oxford University Press.

Vickers, J., Thompson, A., Collins, G. S., Childs, M., and Hain, R. (2007) Place and provision of palliative care for children with progressive cancer: a study by the Paediatric Oncology Nurses' Forum/United Kingdom Children's Cancer Study Group Palliative Care Working Group. *Journal of Clinical Oncology* **25**(28): 4472–6.

Whittle, M. and Cutts, S. (2002) Time to go home: assisting families to take their child home following a planned hospital or hospice death. *Paediatric Nursing* **14**(10): 24–8.

Widger, K., Davies, D., Drouin, D. J., Beaune, L., Daoust, L., Farran, R. P., Humbert, N., Nalewajek, F., Rattray, M., Rugg, M. and Bishop, M. (2007) Pediatric patients receiving palliative care in Canada. *Archives of Pediatrics and Adolescent Medicine* **16**(6): 597–602.

Wolfe, J., Grier, H. E., Klar, N., Levin, S. B., Ellenbogen, J. M., .Salem-Schatz, S., Emanuel, E. J. and Weeks, J. C. (2000) Symptoms and suffering at the end of life in children with cancer. *The New England Journal of Medicine* **342**: 326–33.

Wolfe, J., Klar, N., Grier, H. E., Duncan, J., Salem-Schatz, S., Emanuel, E. J. and Weeks, J. C. (2000) Understanding of prognosis among parents of children who died of cancer. *Journal of the American Medical Association* **284**(19): 2469–75.

WHO (World Health Organization) (1998) *Cancer Pain Relief and Palliative Care in Children*. Geneva: WHO.

WHO (World Health Organization) (2004) *The Solid Facts: Palliative Care*, Davies, E. and Higginson, I. J. (eds). Geneva: WHO.

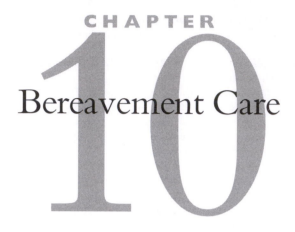

Bereavement Care

Jenni Thomas OBE and Ann Chalmers

Introduction

The death of a child has been described as the ultimate tragedy (Rando 1986, Riches and Dawson 1996). No parent ever expects their child to die before they do (Rowa-Dewar 2002) and their grief is for a whole future of hopes and dreams that will never be fulfilled (Laakso and Paunonen-Ilmonen 2001). When families have a child with a life-limiting condition, they experience loss – and therefore grief – from the point of diagnosis. Parents often say that even though their child's death is anticipated, when their child actually dies the experience is profoundly shocking. For parents, the agony of losing a child at any age is unparalleled (Wilson 1988, Rallison and Moules 2004). The feelings have been described by parents as being similar to an amputation, with a vital part of themselves missing (Klass 1988).

Working with families whose child has died and being faced with the enormity of their loss is one of the most difficult things any professional has to face. Being with families who are grieving is challenging and emotionally demanding, requiring a particular quality of response and support for each member of the interdisciplinary team. While there have undoubtedly been significant advances in paediatric palliative medicine, it is not always possible to ensure that all suffering will be relieved, and professionals are acutely aware of how vividly families remember events surrounding the death of their child (Wolfe *et al.* 2000). Home is often the preferred setting for end-of-life care for many children, young people and their families (Vickers and Carlisle 2000, Hynson and Sawyer 2001 Brook 2006). It is essential at the end of life, wherever the location, to ensure good communication between the family and those involved in their care (This is discussed in Chapters 3 and 9).

Poor bereavement care can exacerbate and prolong families' distress; while care that is sensitive and appropriate can help families in their grief. Our ability to be human, genuine and caring is what makes the difference. Families say the effects of such support are positive and enduring (Thomas 2007).

As policy endorses bereavement support as an essential element of palliative care (ACT and RCPCH 2003, DH 2008) this chapter looks at grief reactions for parents and family members following the death of a child. In addition, it examines ways in which to support families, and encourages an examination of professionals' own values and beliefs about death and dying in order that parents receive the best possible bereavement care available.

KEY POINT

The death of a child evokes different reactions in parents, and for each parent, grieving is an individualized process.

Anticipatory grief

ACT and RCPCH (2003) identify how bereavement support for many of these families may be needed prior to the death, especially for those who have no treatment options available, or for those with multiple bereavements. It is essential to recognize that families may have already begun their grieving process before their child has died.

Anticipatory grief has been a widely debated phenomenon in health and social care literature. Anticipatory grief describes the mix of emotions that can be experienced when living in expectation of an impending loss. This type of grief was first identified by Lindemann (1944) in relatives of soldiers returning from service in the Second World War. Some of these families had lived for many years with the potential loss of their loved one and greeted them on return with apparent coldness, having undergone some type of adjustment and grieving in advance. Kübler-Ross (1970) used the term 'preparatory grief', referring to the grief that the terminally ill patient has to undergo in order to prepare him/herself for the final separation from this world; 'anticipatory grief' has been utilized when referring to the care of children with malignancies (Binger *et al.* 1969). Binger *et al.* concluded that the time of diagnosis was often equated with death for families with a child who had cancer, and it was at that point that grieving commenced. Moreover, findings from a study by Seecharan *et al.* (2004) indicated that mothers who experienced the sudden death of a child experienced a more intensive grief reaction than those who had a child that died from a chronic condition. This further supports the notion of a degree of anticipatory grief, where parents may find there is an opportunity to prepare psychologically for the death of their child. Brown (2007) identified that anticipatory grief seems to accelerate over time, in contrast to grief after bereavement, which usually decelerates slowly with the passage of time.

From the point that a family receives the information that their child will be receiving end-of-life care, sensitive support based on their individual needs is vital through this difficult time. Parents are likely to oscillate between periods of acceptance and denial in trying to take in the enormity of what they have been told. It is often difficult for anyone to predict with certainty the trajectory of a child's illness, or to be precise about when the child will actually die, and parents often experience a rollercoaster journey through refusal to believe the diagnosis, raised hopes and despair.

During this time, when parents are grieving in anticipation of their child's death, feelings often go unexpressed as they try to remain strong for their child, for each other and for their other children. The dawning realization that their child will die can plunge parents into many of the symptoms and emotions that are commonly experienced after a death has happened, including shock, anger, denial, guilt, deep sadness, helplessness, powerlessness, physical and emotional pain, changes in eating and sleeping patterns, and depression.

Anticipatory grieving can also be the route to parents beginning to accept the reality of what is to come, and for some it affords them the opportunity to face that reality and be able to say and do some of the things they would wish to before their child dies.

CLINICAL FOCUS

'We knew Guy was going to die, and I had a lovely lady minister I had met come round to see him weekly for six months, so that at his funeral the Minister taking the funeral would have known him, and wouldn't just be talking about a stranger she had never met.

I talked about his death with him quite openly, and explained how he would be buried, not cremated, as I needed a headstone and grave to visit. He was quite practical about all of this and it was my husband and I who broke down, but never Guy. He told me he never wanted me to forget him. As if I could.'

Micki. From Chalmers (2008) with permission from the Child Bereavement Trust.

For the dying child, there is likely to be a strong need to protect other family members, so the child's feelings about his or her impending death may go unexpressed. If the adults around can help them, the child or young person may want to make known their wishes for their funeral and after their death – what they would like to wear, whether they would like to be buried or cremated, who they would like to receive their special possessions and so on. There may also be things they might like to write or draw for people before they die.

ACTIVITY

Consider how you would feel, engaging in such activities with a dying child or young person, and what might you need to consider, both for the child and for yourself.

Working with bereaved families

All professionals, of whatever discipline, who come into contact with grieving families have a role to play in bereavement care. The smallest act may mean so much to a bereaved family. A study by MacDonald *et al.* (2005) reported how parents greatly value and appreciate receiving cards, as well as efforts from staff to telephone or attend the funeral.

The key worker (discussed in Chapter 2) has been identified as the person who will ensure that bereavement support following the death is carried out by someone with appropriate training (ACT and RCPCH 2003). It is normal in the first instance that the interdisciplinary team decides who is to provide the bereavement follow-up. This is usually someone who has been involved in the child's care and knows the family well.

Beardsmore and Fitzmaurice (2002) assert that families may require more formal counselling if they display signs of dysfunctional or complicated grief. ACT and RCPCH (2003) stipulate that a health or social care professional who has a close therapeutic relationship with the family is in the best position to assess specific needs in bereavement, and should be able to identify those bereaved parents who require more specialist support. Thomas (1994) suggests that, if further help is required, it can also be useful if it is provided by someone who has not previously been involved with the family. Other families may request this type of intervention, and in either case should be directed towards agencies that provide this type of service.

ACTIVITY

Consider which members of the interdisciplinary team in your place of work provide bereavement support for families.

A common area of concern and uncertainty for professionals is knowing what to say to bereaved families. It is a real skill to be able to bear the distress and pain with the family, recognizing that being there and often not saying much at all is enormously important.

ACTIVITY

In what situations have you found it most difficult to listen and talk to families in distress? Can you think what might have helped?

Very often, as carers, we fear that we will make the situation worse. Instinctively, people who choose a caring profession do so because they want to take pain away and make things better. Families attending Child Bereavement Charity (CBC) support groups tell us that the worst has happened and the only thing that makes anything worse is when someone diminishes their loss by trying to make it better. Every family and situation is unique. Knowing what to say comes with understanding, experience and a certain amount of trusting our intuition.

If we have been able to see the world through the families' eyes, it is likely that they will know we care even if we sometimes make mistakes in what we say. As Burnard (1992) describes, the intuitive dimension tends to be undervalued and yet health care professionals are often required to be intuitive and guess what other people are feeling in order to empathize with them.

Developing self-awareness

Part of becoming self-aware entails discovering and exploring the emotional dimension. Health care professionals must deal with other people's emotions and there is a positive link between the way in which we handle our own emotions and the way in which we handle those of others. If we understand and can appropriately express our own anger, fear, grief and embarrassment, we will be better able to handle them in other people. In caring for others, we must get to know ourselves better (Burnard 1997).

When we have chosen to work with families facing loss, it is important as professionals to take into account our own needs and attitudes to death and dying. Reflecting on and being aware of our own reactions to situations of bereavement help us to understand better our strengths and weaknesses, and will support our ability to work effectively with grieving families. Reflecting on our own life experiences can help us to recognize our responses and ways of coping when facing situations of loss.

This reflection may also help us to identify areas that we ourselves may not have fully resolved, and also to recognize the potential for reactions to our own losses to be triggered when we come into contact with someone who is experiencing something similar.

The way we are will fundamentally affect the care we offer to families. So in working with grieving people, it is essential that we become self-aware, identify our own strengths and weaknesses, and recognize our own needs. This will enable us to be better prepared for the demanding situations we face when working with bereaved families. Developing self-awareness allows us to understand how we think and feel, and enables us to clarify our values and beliefs. Supporting ourselves has to begin with self-awareness, which is not simply about knowing what has happened to us in our lives – whether personally or professionally – but also about acknowledging the impact of those life experiences on us and recognizing how they may even affect the way we are and how we work.

=========================== **ACTIVITY** ===========================

Reflecting on your own childhood, can you identify what influence this might have had on you and your work?

Coming close to families who are grieving, we need to be mindful that any hurts and losses we have experienced in our own lives may be brought to the surface, even though we may feel we have dealt with them, whether in our personal or working lives. Grief is contagious – our emotions will often mirror those of the families we are supporting. Families value professionals who are able to show their feelings; however, it is important that we remind ourselves that, however much we care, we cannot know their pain.

Working with grieving families may well bring up feelings about our own experiences of being a child, the parenting (or lack of parenting) we received, and how we feel about children – whether the children we have, the children we may hope to have in the future, or the children we perhaps might not have been able to have, for whatever reason.

Working with families after a child has died is likely to put us in touch with our own feelings and concerns about loss and death, so it is little wonder that this is immensely challenging work that often leaves professionals feeling inadequate and helpless as well as humbled and privileged to be with the family at such an important time.

Everyone needs a sense of purpose in life, something that gives their life meaning. For some people this comes through a religious conviction, whereas others may be driven by political or philosophical beliefs. It is important to explore our own beliefs and motivations, and to recognize and acknowledge that not everyone thinks about things the same way as we do. This means recognizing the judgements and assumptions we tend to make, which may get in the way of fully caring for a grieving family. If we are clear about what we believe, it will be easier to be open to what other people believe, even if we do not agree with them.

Many of us choose not to think about our own deaths, and actively avoid the subject. But if we are to deal with death in our working lives and help bereaved families, we need to confront our own fears and limitations about the subject. Being aware of how we feel and what we think can help towards a greater understanding of the families we care for.

ACTIVITY

Think about your own mortality. What would you like your epitaph to be?

In looking at diverse cultural needs in bereavement, it is helpful to recognize that each of us comes from a different culture, the culture of our family, the family in which we grew up. The attitudes our family holds about death and dying may well be very different from what we experience in our work. This can be challenging for us as professionals; however, by having an understanding of ourselves and identifying our feelings and needs as being separate from those of the families we care for, we shall be better able help them do what is right for them rather than advising them solely according to what we think.

As professionals, we work with people from a variety of cultures, and it is helpful to look at our sensitivity towards those who are culturally different and to develop our self-awareness (Burnard 1997). When interacting with people from different backgrounds, cultures and faiths, it is particularly important to ask them about their beliefs, and what is likely to be of help and support to them at the time of bereavement, and, just as important, what might be considered insensitive at that time. Through CBC support groups we learn continually from families and can therefore find new ways in which to support them. Bereaved families can feel as if they are in a foreign country, with no language and no map, and the power of being fully heard cannot be underestimated.

Listening to bereaved families

Listening has been identified as an essential skill within children's palliative care (Rushton 2005). A good listener helps people to listen to themselves. Learning how to listen effectively is a fundamental element in bereavement care (Cook 1999).

The component parts of the Chinese pictogram for 'listening' graphically illustrates how fully engaged we need to be in order to truly listen (see Figure 10.1). Being able to communicate and listen effectively and appropriately enables us to help and support bereaved people usefully and safely. Listening to a family's individual needs, anxieties and beliefs enables us to meet them on their own ground; and help them to express the meaning this loss holds for them.

We need to listen with our ears, attending to the words, the tone of voice and the feelings being conveyed. We need to listen with our eyes, observing body language and facial expressions; maintaining regular eye contact lets the other person know we are concentrating on their words. We need to give our undivided attention to the other person and notice not only what is being said but equally what is not being spoken. By setting time boundaries at the outset, we create a safe environment and enable the other person to know how long they can expect us to spend with them, so that the interaction does not come to an abrupt end.

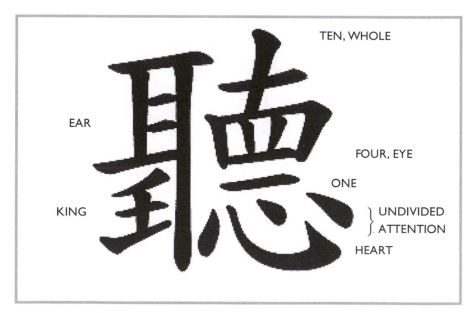

Figure 10.1 Chinese pictogram meaning 'listening'

Source: Adapted from Child Bereavement Charity course material 'When a child dies – supporting parents and family members', with the kind permission of CBC

We need to listen with our heart, communicating our interest and empathy by our own verbal intonation and body language, and we need to use all of ourselves to connect with the other person, to ensure that there is genuine two-way communication. In all of this we need to listen with great respect – as depicted in the 'king' symbol of the pictogram – the respect that should be afforded to a king.

Active listening requires that the professional is truly self-aware, and has explored and found ways to manage his or her own feelings. If we consciously make time to listen to ourselves and can bear to confront our innermost feelings, then we are more available to focus on others without our own feelings getting in the way and taking us away from the person we are listening to.

Working with bereaved, distressed and anxious families, there may be times when we find it hard to really listen to them – simply not having an appropriate place to talk without fear of interruption can make listening very difficult, for example. Sometimes, what is being implied, what is being avoided by bereaved parents, or what is not being said, is significant. All these subtle communications will be more readily noticeable if we focus totally on the person we are listening to. We may also find that a spontaneous response comes to mind more readily when we listen fully and allow ourselves to take in what is being said to us. This often lessens anxiety about 'What can I say in response to this?' Not saying anything does not mean we have not heard, and sometimes the need to speak is ours. Silence can be golden.

Listening carefully leads to more effective communication. The death of a child cannot be 'fixed', and we cannot provide families with a solution to their grief; but a genuine, congruent response that is accepting of what they feel and think will help them come to an understanding for themselves. Often, when interacting with other people, it is tempting to try and to solve their problems, to tell them what to do, how they feel and to make their decisions for them. It is much harder to acknowledge that individuals have the capacity to know best about their own feelings and actions, and empower them to make decisions for themselves. When we are preparing to say something in response or are trying to give advice, we are in danger of finding ourselves waiting for our chance to speak rather than listening to what the other person is really saying. Anger may sometimes be a significant part of an individual's grief. If as a professional we feel we are being attacked and accused, it can be very difficult to listen. The natural reaction is to become defensive, but if we can help the family to explore the anger without trying to rationalize or justify it, they are more likely to feel heard and understood.

ACTIVITY

How do you instinctively respond to another person's anger? Consider whether there are ways in which you might respond more helpfully?

Pressures of other work, insufficient time, tiredness and our personal feelings can all make active listening difficult; however, with time, we can consciously develop this important skill.

To facilitate this, Carl Rogers (1991) considers that three core attitudes are necessary:

- *Empathic listening* – this is very hard to do, and involves giving our full attention to the person speaking by putting to one side our own thoughts, so we can concentrate on what the person is saying. If we can let the other person feel that we are really listening and have understood what has been said, then the individual is more likely to open up and entrust us with personal and private feelings. Blocks to empathy include thinking we know best and wanting to solve problems for others.

- *Acceptance* – we need to be able to accept whatever is said without being judgemental or critical. This can be difficult, as our own prejudices and conditioning may intrude, but it is important in to allowing the other person to feel safe and able to explore issues more deeply.

- *To be genuine and congruent* – this requires us to be honest and open in order to promote trust in the person we are listening to. A false attitude will soon be picked up and can destroy the relationship we are building.

The process of grieving

> If bereavement is a wound, then grief is the inflammation that follows. It causes pain, swelling and disturbance of function. It can last a long time and may leave scars. Yet, it is the process by which healing occurs (Wilson 1991).

Grief is experienced by the whole family – parents, siblings and the wider family circle. The experience will be felt uniquely by each individual (Rowa-Dewar 2002) but there are universal traits.

=== **ACTIVITY** ===

List the factors you think influence the outcome of bereavement for families.

Worden (1991) stresses that mourning – the emotional process that occurs after a loss – is an essential and necessarily painful healing process, which is achieved through a series of tasks. The word 'task' implies work, and grieving is very hard work; however, accomplishing these tasks is the route to greater psychological strength and growth. Failure to complete the tasks can lead to complicated grief where people become stuck and unable to move forward. The tasks are not necessarily achieved in any particular order or one at a time – people will go in and out of the tasks as they struggle to understand what has happened on an intellectual and emotional level, and to find an appropriate place in their lives for the person who has died. Intellectual recognition tends to come first, and sometimes relatively quickly, whereas the emotional recognition takes longer and will be worked through alongside the other tasks.

Accepting the reality

Initially, the bereaved person may be in a state of shock, even when a death has been anticipated. This can be manifested as an outpouring of emotion, or the antithesis may be seen, with the person displaying no emotion at all, appearing very controlled, calm and detached. This task recognizes the need for them to intellectually recognize the reality of the loss they have experienced.

Some people may not immediately be able to acknowledge what has happened and may cope by denying it or refusing to talk about it. Being able to see the dead person, being involved as much as possible in the preparations for the funeral, and observing rituals and traditions, all assist in facing the reality. Families need to be supported in following the mourning rituals appropriate to their culture and beliefs. How able the dying person and their family were to face the reality of the impending death will have a significant bearing on how they are emotionally after the death. Coming to a gradual acceptance of the death allows the family to begin the long and difficult task of adjustment.

Experiencing the pain or emotional aspects of the loss

As the reality of the loss is recognized intellectually, the pain of grief begins to be felt. This involves a bewildering mixture of powerful emotions that need to be allowed, identified for what they are, and fully experienced (Laakso and Paunonen-Ilmonen 2001).

As the numbed feeling gradually subsides and the reality of what has happened begins to be experienced, the bereaved person may at times feel a range of intensely painful emotions. These get in they way of everything they think and do. Their grief may overwhelm them, so they are preoccupied with how they feel and incapable of thinking about anything else. It is natural in grief to have a diminished capacity to think very readily of others, and to be more self-absorbed than usual. They may overreact to other people's comments and appear irritable. A writer and a bereaved mother, eloquently described her extreme sensitivity as feeling as though she had 'one skin less'.

As well as extreme sadness, the bereaved often experience guilt, anger and resentment. Many people struggle with guilt about some aspect of their relationship with the dead person. Perhaps they had left unsaid their true feelings, or said things they did not really mean. Maybe they had not spent enough time with them, or really listened. If there has been denial that the death would happen – either on the part of the terminally ill person or their family members – things might have gone unspoken and people can then be stuck in with feelings of guilt and regret for a long time.

Feelings of anger can be extremely powerful. The bereaved person may feel anger towards the dead person; anger for the loss of control that death brings; anger at the medical team for not curing the illness, keeping the dead person alive, or being denied the type of death they would have wanted for that person; and anger at God for letting it happen. They may feel resentment towards a family member who may not have behaved in a way that was expected.

KEY POINT

Expression of feelings is an essential part of the grieving process and requires the sympathetic presence of a caring, supportive person.

Grief is not a mental illness, though sleeplessness, anxiety, fear, anger and a preoccupation with self can all add up to a feeling of 'going mad'. These feelings are natural, and when experienced and expressed will become less frequent and begin to subside over time. Talking about them and bringing them into the open is helpful. Expressing grief is cathartic, and attempts to short- circuit these feelings rarely help in the long term and may cause deep-seated problems in the years ahead. If grief is denied, or anger and guilt persist to the exclusion of other feelings, help may be required from a professional counsellor.

Adjusting to the new reality

Loss inevitably brings change, which will vary in nature and degree depending on the significance of the loss. The work is in accepting the inevitable changes and finding appropriate ways to manage them in what will be a changed life. Facing life without someone important to you is an extremely difficult and painful process; for parents who have experienced the death of their child, this can be a life-long process. No one can fill the aching void their child has left, and each day brings constant reminders of their child's absence. The future may seem uncertain or even frightening, and a tremendous effort is required just to get through every day. It may take many months before the bereaved person is able to dwell less on the sad events surrounding the death and starts to function more as they once did, although they will be inevitably be changed.

To find a place in your life for the person who has died, and find ways to remember them

This stage, according to Worden, involves moving on to a new way of life without the person who has died, while holding on to important memories of them. It is not about forgetting or ceasing to love the person, but about finding ways to remember him or her that allow you to continue with life – a changed life. It is a way of reinvesting in life again – which can often feel like a betrayal – but that still allows that person to be remembered in a less painful way.

This is perhaps the most difficult task of all. Bereaved parents need to find a place for their child within them emotionally, so that they can take their memories of their child forward with them into the future, but in a way that allows them to continue with life rather than keeping them in the pain of their loss. There is a sense of being able ultimately to put the acute sadness aside and look to the future, while recalling happy memories of the child who has died, and finding comfort and pleasure in those memories. It is also a way of making life more meaningful and winning back some control, so that the bereaved person is not continually trapped in painful memories.

It is normal at anniversaries and other significant times (such as when their child would have started school, gone to college, had children of their own and so on) for the very painful initial feelings of grief to be aroused again for a time.

ACTIVITY

Consider your experience of the tasks of mourning in relation to a family you have supported, and in relation to a loss you have experienced yourself.

Worden's model focuses very much on working through emotions in relation to loss, but subsequent research papers suggest a more sociologically-based model, recognizing the desire in the bereaved typically to want to talk about the person who has died, and to talk to others who knew that person. Together, principally through conversation, they construct a story that places the dead within their lives, a story capable of enduring through time, that integrates the memory of the person into their ongoing lives. The process therefore involves moving on with, as well as without, the person who has died (Walter 1996). Similarly, Klass *et al.* (1996) acknowledge that there is a continuing bond and ongoing relationship between bereaved parents and their dead child, a bond that is not broken by the fact of death. The notion of 'continuing bonds' recognizes parental grief as a means of trying to maintain a connection with their dead child (Davies 2004). Parents need to find a way of integrating their dead child into their lives and an appropriate emotional place for that child, which helps them maintain a sense of their child's presence in everyday life, but in a way that is different from when the child was alive.

FURTHER READING

Read Davies, R. (2004) New understandings of parental grief: literature review, *Journal of Advanced Nursing* **46**(5): 506–13.

Consider how this could apply to your work with families who have lost a child.

Bereaved parents do not stop parenting – parental instincts do not simply die with the child. This can, however, create a particular challenge for health care professionals, who need to help families end their relationship with the professionals in an appropriate and helpful way. Bearing in mind the enormous emotional energy that families invest in professionals who have shared a deeply meaningful journey with them, they may never think that there will be an ending to the relationship.

However, it is crucial that we keep in sight that there does need to be an ending with the family at some point in time, and not to confuse the family by offering friendship, because this is usually offered without limit of time. All families should be offered an equitable service and we need to support ourselves by being mindful to maintain appropriate professional boundaries.

Setting boundaries enables us to maintain a separateness that contains and holds both the family and ourselves, and is vitally important if we are to work safely in this field. Being mindful of what belongs to us emotionally and what belongs to those we care for in our work, and giving thought to where we set our own limits in terms of what we're prepared to offer, is essential in establishing clear boundaries. When adequate boundaries are not put in place, there is the potential for us to be 'sucked in' more than might be good for either ourselves or the family; we may then be tempted to take over rather than empower and support people to manage things for themselves. The truth is that, for most of us, it can be very seductive to be needed! It is crucial to have this in our awareness, and to find support for what we might struggle with in this respect.

ACTIVITY

Think of the boundaries you put in place around your work with families. In what circumstances are these most likely to be challenged?

Grief is a solitary and isolating experience (Bucaro *et al.* 2005). Even when others in the family are grieving, each parent can feel alone. Couples often have an inability to communicate with one another and to express the awfulness of their feelings (Feeley and Gottlieb 1988). A mother's response to the death of a child is frequently different from that of the father (Feeley and Gottlieb 1988). Mothers' behaviour tends to be loss-orientated, and they are very much concerned with their feelings. When a child has died they need memories on which to focus their grief and have a need to talk about what has happened and how they feel (Laakso and Paunonen-Ilmonen 2001). In contrast, fathers' behaviour tends to be more restoration-orientated, wishing to 'fix' what is wrong and look to the future. These different ways of dealing with grief can put a significant strain on the parents' relationship and it is helpful for them to understand that their partner's response to grief is natural, and to find ways of sharing their feelings and reaching out to one another (Lang and Gottlieb 1993).

KEY POINT

Mothers and fathers need support in bereavement. Gender differences in grief reactions are apparent.

Stroebe and Schut (1999) proposed a dual model of grieving in which people engage in both loss-orientated and restoration-orientated grieving activity, oscillating between the two reactions (see Figure 10.2). This may be particularly true when families are living through the peaks and troughs of hope and despair so often associated with terminal illness.

When people engage in either activity to the exclusion of the other it can cause difficulties. Women need help to develop some form of restorative response to

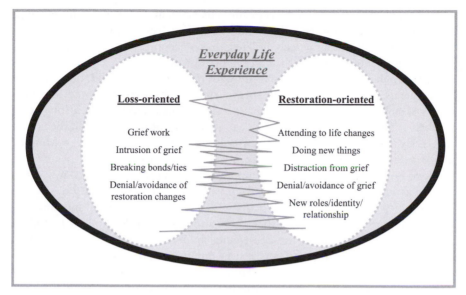

Figure 10.2 A dual process model of coping with bereavement

Source: Stroebe and Schut (1999). Reproduced with the kind permission of Professor Stroebe.

enable them to move on from the intensity of the pain, and men need to be helped to allow themselves to face up to and explore their painful feelings.

Professionals may also experience this oscillation for themselves, and recognize how their behaviour – and that of their colleagues – may differ depending on whether they are focused on loss or restoration at that particular time. As with couples, we as carers may judge and misinterpret the behaviour of colleagues when it is different from our own, and need to be mindful that the behaviour exhibited at work may well not be how they manage their feelings away from the work environment.

ACTIVITY

Consider a personal experience of loss that you have had. Write down examples of when you exhibited loss-orientated behaviour, and when you were able to be more restorative. Now consider a work-related experience of loss. How did you behave then? How did your colleagues behave?

Siblings

Siblings are central to the family unit and form their own subsystem (Sourkes *et al.* (2005). A study by Lauer *et al.* (1985) interviewed thirty-six children/young people between the ages of 5 and 26 years who had lost a brother or sister less than one year before participating in the study. Here, the significant anguish caused to siblings if they are excluded from death–related events was postulated.

It also identified how children whose sibling had died in the home felt more aware and better supported by parents. If children do not feel involved it can create a situation where the sibling feels isolated, misconceptions are formed and ultimately there is interference in the bereavement process.

Bereaved parents must cope not only with the loss of their child, but also with the demands of everyday life and their surviving children. The way in which bereaved siblings are parented will have a significant impact on their long-term wellbeing, but bereaved parents' ability to parent the other children in the family effectively is likely to have been compromised for at least a time, both during the dying child's illness and after his or her death.

How parents and professionals respond emotionally to brothers and sisters when a child is dying can have a profound effect on a sibling's ability to manage the enormity of what is happening. As with adults, children need information, and the opportunity to express their fears and questions (Stokes 2004). Often, with the best of intentions, the adults and children in the family protect each other from painful feelings and experiences; but it is impossible not to communicate with children (Monroe 1995), and not speaking only serves to create fear, confusion and anxiety rather than to diminish it, sometimes leading to a conspiracy of silence.

Having a sick brother or sister who then dies can give rise to a complex mix of emotions and behaviour in siblings (Giovanola 2005). Their life may have been dominated by anxious and distant parents, hospital stays and not feeling as important as the child who is poorly. There may be strong feelings of resentment and jealousy at the attention that has been given to a sick child, or there may be feelings of relief that the death has happened, and they will have their parents all to themselves again. Siblings may also experience tremendous guilt in entertaining these negative feelings. Sometimes a child may have wished their brother or sister would die, and need overt reassurance afterwards that the death was not their fault.

Often siblings may not be able to express themselves through words, but what they are experiencing can be reflected in their behaviour. Children often regress in grief, perhaps needing more cuddles and physical affection; bedwetting and violent outbursts that seem to come from nowhere are sometimes symptoms of their grief. Alternatively, they may not show any feelings at all. They may have spent years anticipating the death of their brother or sister, so that when it happens, they exhibit less sadness than their parents might have expected. Children tend to oscillate between loss and restoration much more naturally than do adults. They tend not to stay sad for very long, but rather to dip in and out of their grief.

WEB LINKS

Go to www.childbereavement.org.uk and www.winstonswish.org.uk

Identify the resources that could be used when working with bereaved children. Consider ways in which these could be used in your workplace.

How children respond to a loss depends on a number of factors: their age and consequent understanding of death; the nature of their relationship with the

I am: relates to personality features which can be strengthened by support but cannot be created.

I have: relates to family and external support structures which can be both provided and strengthened.

I can: relates to a child's own social and interpersonal, skills which must be learnt and can be taught.

Figure 10.3 Resilience model

Source: Grotberg (1995).

person who has died; the circumstances of the death; the reactions of other family members to the death; the overall effect on the family unit; and their culture and religion.

Children tend to be helped greatly when their natural resilience is supported. This relates closely to their self-esteem, which is nurtured when children feel included in what is happening. The factors that contribute to a child's resilience are described in Figure 10.3.

Looking after ourselves

> Progress in palliation includes not only looking after children but also looking after the staff who care for these children and their families (Baverstock and Finlay 2006a: 774).

This quotation highlights that providing palliative care for children and families, and support for professionals in their caring role, are inextricably linked. Providing palliative care for children can be stressful (Maunder 2006) and can present the interdisciplinary team with a range of emotional challenges. However, team members can find caring for a dying child and his or her family to be something that yields them profound satisfaction as well as being a source of great pain (Rushton 2005). While considerable progress has been made in paediatric end-of-life care, the impact of this work on professional carers has received far less attention. Parkes (1998) acknowledges that grief is a natural reaction for those working with the dying. The death of a child may also evoke feelings of failure in professionals and weakness in the face of incurable illnesses (Hynson *et al.* 2003).

The key to managing the feelings this work engenders in us is self-awareness. Just as with children, we need to nurture our ability to be resilient. To do this, we need to be able to read our own signs of distress and find ways to make time for ourselves. One of the reasons that people burn out in caring professions is that they often do not notice they are under pressure until it is too late. When looking after bereaved families, we may carry feelings of discomfort in our bodies – and we need to listen to the messages our bodies send us. All too often we desensitize ourselves and ignore signs that we are under ever-increasing stress. Very often when we feel unable to deal with our own emotions, we develop protective strategies, such as distancing ourselves from the emotions of others, appearing unaffected and detached, or conversely becoming very busy in order to avoid the pain. When we do not take care of ourselves we can begin to develop negative feelings about ourselves and our work, and see ourselves as failures.

This may develop into cynicism, anger and resentment, which can have an impact on both our family and professional relationships. Some of the warning signs of feeling depleted include experiencing chronic exhaustion, frequently being upset, having difficulty eating or sleeping, developing headaches or backaches, having nightmares, feeling worthless and pessimistic, avoiding contact with others, leaving work early and arriving late, or perhaps overworking.

ACTIVITY

Consider the ways in which staff can receive support in your practice area.

It is essential to take the time to seek support from colleagues and others when we need it. A variety of support strategies can assist health and social care professionals manage stress in caring for dying children and their families (Liben *et al.* 2008).

Factors that have been recognized as helpful in supporting ourselves include: acknowledging and understanding our own emotions and having somewhere safe to express them; having training in understanding ourselves in relation to this work, and in understanding families' needs in grief and loss; being clear about the boundaries of our role; being part of a supportive team; and having access to regular support and supervision where we feel able to be honest and open about how this work affects us (Michelson and Steinhorn 2007).

A study by Baverstock and Finlay (2006b) examined the staff support offered in children's hospices in the UK. All the hospices that replied (n = 26) indicated they had access to a bereavement counsellor, which staff found invaluable. Other support networks highlighted through the study embraced a comprehensive induction programme for staff including the opportunity to consider self awareness and grief, loss and anticipatory grief as well as team-building days and social activities.

The role of the manager is vital in creating an environment in which such issues can be addressed openly and effectively. Staff debriefing and reflection is important within the interdisciplinary team. A model such as McNeilly *et al.* (2006) can be used for this purpose, and its value in structuring debriefing has been recognized (DHSSPS 2008). Training and education is vital for staff who support bereaved families; courses such as those run by the Child Bereavement Charity can provide an excellent support network for the professionals as well as teaching them self- management, coping skills and boundary strategies.

Equally important is having personal coping mechanisms, and these will vary from person to person (Michelson and Steinhorn 2007). They may include laughter, relaxation, exercise, alternative therapies and doing things we enjoy. All contribute to our sense of wellbeing, and, of course, to that elusive work/life balance. Acknowledging our own need for support and doing something about it is a strength, not a weakness, and developing relationships that will support us and be a resource when we need help for ourselves will ultimately enable us to be resilient in this work.

━━━━━━━━━━━━━━━━━━━━━━ **ACTIVITY** ━━━━━━━━━━━━━━━━━━━━━━

Consider the personal coping mechanisms you use to look after yourself.

Conclusion

This chapter opened with the acknowledgement that the death of a child clearly defies the natural expected order of life events, and leads to a deep sense of loss and grief for the parents and the whole family circle. The fact that grief is a very individualized and extremely painful experience for parents has also been highlighted. The challenges faced by families who have suffered the loss of a child have been examined, alongside the acknowledgement that helping families face the enormity of their loss is one of the most difficult things any professional has to manage. When we have chosen to work with families facing loss, it is important as professionals to take into account our own needs and attitudes to death and dying, and to develop our self-awareness in relation to this challenging area of work. As grief is such a uniquely personal experience, a co-ordinated and individualized approach to bereavement care is essential, where each member of the family is supported, including mothers and fathers, siblings, grandparents and the wider family. Palliative care does not end when the child dies, and the interdisciplinary team must assist and support the family as they negotiate the complexities of adjusting to life without their child. Bereavement care must therefore be an integral part of quality care provision.

Key resources

Chalmers, A. (ed.) (2008) *Farewell, My Child*. West Wycombe: Child Bereavement Charity.
Child Bereavement Charity resources can be found at: www.childbereavement.org
Worden, J. W. (1991) *Grief Counselling and Grief Therapy: A Handbook for the Mental Health Practitioner* (2nd edn). London: Springer.

CHAPTER SUMMARY

- Families experience loss, and therefore grief, from the point of diagnosis.

- The death of a child leads to a deep and long-lasting grief.

- Families have very individualized needs in bereavement – there is no right way to grieve and families do as they must in grief.

- Siblings also have specific needs in bereavement.

- The essence of effective support is based on appropriate and sensitive communication.

- Our greatest learning comes from listening to families and being open to reflecting on the impact of this work on us as professionals.

- Bereavement care is a key component of palliative care.

References

ACT and RCPCH (Association for Children with Life-threatening or Terminal Conditions and their Families and Royal College of Paediatrics and Child Health) (2003) A Guide to the Development of Children's Palliative Care Services 2nd edn. Bristol: ACT.

Baverstock, A. and Finlay, F. (2006a) Specialist registrars' emotional responses to a patient's death. *Archives of Disease in Childhood* **91**: 774–6.

Baverstock, A. and Finlay, F. (2006b) A study of staff support mechanisms within children's hospices. *International Journal of Palliaitive Nursing* **12**(11): 506–8.

Beardsmore, S. and Fitzmaurice, N. (2002) Palliaitve care in paediatric oncology. *European Journal of Cancer* **38**: 1900–7.

Binger, C. M., Ablin, A. R., Feuerstein, M. D., Kushner, J. H., Zoger, S. and Mikkelsen, C. (1969) Childhood leukemia: emotional impact on patient and family. *New England Journal of Medicine* **280**: 414–18.

Brook, L. (2006) Developing the Liverpool integrated pathway for the dying child. Presentation at the 3rd International Paediatric Palliative Care Conference, Cardiff, 21–23 June.

Brown, E. (2007) *Supporting the Child and the Family in Paediatric Palliative Care.* London: Jessica Kingsley.

Bucaro, P. J., Asher, L. M., and Miles Curry, D. (2005) Bereavement care: one children's hospital's compassionate plan for parents and families. *Journal of Emergency Nursing* **31**: 305–8.

Burnard, P. (1992) *Effective Communication Skills for Health Professionals.* London: Chapman & Hall.

Burnard, P. (1997) Know yourself. *A Manual of Self Awareness Activities.* London: Whurr.

Chalmers, A. (ed.) (2008) *Farewell, My Child.* West Wycombe: Child Bereavement Charity.

Cook, P. (1999) *Supporting Sick Children and Their Families.* London: Balliere Tindall.

Davies, R. (2004) New understandings of parental grief: literature review, *Journal of Advanced Nursing* **46**(5): 506–13.

DH (Department of Health) (DH) (2008) *Better Care: Better Lives. Improving outcomes and experiences for children, young people and their families living with life-limiting and life-threatening conditions.* London: Department of Health.

DHSSPS (Department of Health, Social Services and Public Safety) (2008) *Integrated Care Pathway for Children and Young People with Complex Physical Healthcare Needs* (Consultation document). Belfast: DHSSPS.

Feeley, N. and Gottlieb, L. N. (1988) Parents' communication and coping following their infant's death. *Omega* **19**(1): 51–67.

Giovanola, J. (2005) Sibling involvement at the end of life. *Journal of Pediatric Oncology Nursing* **22**(4): 222–6.

Grotberg, E. (1995) *A Guide to Promoting Resilience in Children.* The Hague: Bernard van Leer Foundation, quoted in Barbnard, P., Morland, I. and Nagy, J. (1999) *Children, Bereavement and Trauma: Nurturing Resilience.* London: Jessica Kingsley, pp. 57–8.

Hynson, J. and Sawyer, S. (2001) Paediatric palliative care: distinctive needs and emerging issues. *Journal of Paediatrics and Child Health* **37**(4): 323–5.

Hynson, J., Gillis, J., Collins, J., Irving, H. and Trethewie, J. (2003) The dying child: how is care different? *Medical Journal of Australia* **179**, S20-S22.

Klass, D. (1988) *Parental Grief, Solace and Resolution.* New York: Springer.

Klass, D., Silverman, P. and Nickman, S. (eds) (1996) *Continuing Bonds: New Understandings of Grief.* London: Taylor & Francis.

Kübler-Ross, E. (1970) *On Death and Dying.* New York: Macmillan.

Laakso, H. and Paunonen-Ilmonen, M. (2001) Mothers' experience of social support following the death of a child. *Journal of Clinical Nursing* **11**: 176–85.

Lang, A. and Gottlieb, L. (1993) Parental grief reactions and marital intimacy following infant death. *Death Studies* **17**: 233–55.

Lauer, M, E., Mulhern, R. K., Bohne, E. B. and Camitta, B. M. (1985) Children's perceptions of their sibling's death at home or hospital: the precursors to differential adjustment. *Cancer Nursing* **8**: 21–7.

Liben, S., Papadatou, D. and Wolfe, J. (2008) Paediatric palliative care: challenges and emerging ideas. *Lancet* **371**(9615): 852–64.

Lindemann, E. (1944) Symptomatology and management of acute grief. *American Journal of Psychiatry* **101**: 141–8.

MacDonald, M.E., Liben, S., Carnevale, F. A., Rennick, J. E.,Wolf, S., Meloche, D. and Cohen, S. R. (2005) Parental perspectives on hospital staff members' acts of kindness and commemoration after a child's death. *Pediatrics* **116**(4): 884–90.

Maunder, E. Z. (2006) Emotion work in the palliaitive nursing care of children and young people. *International Journal of Palliative Nursing* **12**(1): 27–33.

McNeilly P., Price, J. and McCloskey, S. (2006) Reflection in children's palliative care: a model. *European Journal of Palliative Care* **13**(1): 31–4.

Michelson, K. N. and Steinhorn, D. M. (2007) Pediatric end-of-life issues and palliative care. *Clinical Pediatric Emergency Medicine* **8**: 212–19.

Monroe, B. (1995) It is impossible not to communicate – helping the bereaved family. In Smith, S. C. and Pennells, M. (eds) *Interventions with Bereaved Children*. London: Jessica Kingsley.

Parkes, C. M. (1998) Coping with loss: the dying adult. *British Medical Journal,* **316**: 1313–15.

Rallison, L. and Moules, N. (2004) The unspeakable nature of pediatric palliative care:; unveiling many cloaks. *Journal of Family Nursing* **10**(3): 287–301.

Rando, T. (1986) *Parental Loss of a Child*. Champaign, IL: Research Press.

Riches, G. and Dawson, P. (1996) An intimate loneliness: evaluating the impact of a child's death on parental self-identity and marital relationships. *Journal of Family Therapy* **18**: 1–22.

Rogers, C. R. (1991) *Client-centred Therapy*. London: Constable.

Rowa-Dewar, N. (2002) Do interventions make a difference for bereaved parents? A systematic review of controlled studies. *International Journal of Palliative Nursing* **8**(9): 452–7.

Rushton, C. H. (2005) A framework for integrated pediatric palliative care: being with dying. *Journal of Pediatric Nursing* **20**(5): 311–23.

Seecharan, M. P. H., Andresen, E., Norris, K.;, Toce, S. (2004) Parents' assessment of quality care and grief following a child's death. *Archives of Paediatric Adolescent Medicine* **158**: 515–20.

Sourkes, B., Frankel, L., Brown, M., Contro, N., Benitz, W., Case, C., Good, J., Jones, L., Komejan, J,, Modderman-Marshall, J., Reichard, W., Sentivany-Collins, S. and Sunde, C. (2005) Food, toys and love: pediatric palliative care. *Current Problems in Pediatric Adolescent Health Care* **35**: 350–6.

Stokes, J. (2004) *Then, Now and Always*. Cheltenham: Winston's Wish.

Stroebe, M. S. and Schut, H. (1999) The dual process model of coping with bereavement: rationale and descriptions. *Death Studies* **23**(3): 197–224.

Thomas, J. (1994) *Supporting Parents when Their Baby Dies*. West Wycombe: Child Bereavement Charity.

Thomas, J. (2007) The helping relationship with parents of babies who have limited or uncertain life expectancy. In Limbrick, P. (ed.) *Family-centred Support for Children with Disabilities and Special Needs*. Hereford: Interconnections, pp. 23–33.

Vickers, J. and Carlisle, C. (2000) Choices and control; parental experiences in pediatric terminal home care. *Journal of Pediatric Oncology Nursing*. **17**(1): 12–21.

Walter, T. (1996) A new model of grief: bereavement and biography. *Mortality* **1**(1): 7–25.

Wilson, D. (1988) The ultimate loss – the dying child. *Loss Grief and Care* **2**: 125–30.

Wilson, R. (1991) Bereavement: what happens when somebody's baby dies. *Journal of the Association of Chartered Physiotherapists in Obstetrics and Gynaecology* **69**(2): 125–30.

Wolfe, J., Klar, N., Holcombe, E. G., Duncan, J., Salem-Schatz, S., Emanuel, E. J. and Weeks, J. C. (2000) Understanding of prognosis among parents of children who died of cancer – impact on treatment goals and integration of palliative care. *Journal of the American Medical Association* **284**(19): 2469–75.

Worden, J. W. (1991) *Grief Counselling and Grief Therapy: A Handbook for the Mental Health Practitioner* (2nd edn). London: Springer.

11

Future Directions for Children's Palliative Care

Sharon McCloskey and Lizzie Chambers

Introduction

At no previous stage in history have the rights and needs of children been so clearly recognized. Globally, this is underpinned by the United Nations Convention on the Rights of the Child, ratified by 193 countries. Historically, however, the rights of children with life-limiting and life-threatening conditions, alongside children with disabilities or complex healthcare needs, have not been fully acknowledged, partly because they form a small percentage of the population and they have not been seen as a priority. But this is changing. As highlighted previously in this book, the numbers of children with life-limiting conditions is increasing as a result of improvements in medical interventions and technological care (Steele 2000, Hewitt-Taylor 2005). Legislation has enshrined in law the rights of disabled children (Children Act 1989 (England), 1995 (Scotland), and the Children (Northern Ireland) Order 1995; Disability Discrimination Act 1995 and the Special Educational Needs and Disability Act 2001) and a range of government policies have outlined the expected standards for service development and provision, to ensure that all children with life-limiting conditions have the opportunity to reach their potential, regardless of their condition or disability (DH 2004, Welsh Assembly Government 2006, DHSSPS 2007, DH 2008). For children with life-limiting conditions and their families, and for those working in this field, there has never been a more favourable climate in which to harness these opportunities to deliver the 'step change' in service provision that these children and their families need and rightly deserve (DH 2008).

This concluding chapter explores key issues for the future of children's palliative care. It highlights that in many ways this is a positive time for children's palliative care, with a growing recognition of the distinct needs of children with life–limiting conditions and their families, and an emerging national and international policy agenda. Core issues for future development are examined, while likely challenges are acknowledged. The reader is encouraged to reflect on these issues in their own practice and to identify ways through which they can make a personal and positive impact to the development of children's palliative care in their own area.

Refining the language of children's palliative care

As discussed in Chapter 1, the terminology of children's palliative care is often ambiguous and confusing. At the time of writing, most policy-makers and those responsible for commissioning services are only just beginning to develop an understanding of children's palliative care. The establishment of a common voice through the clarification of a common language is vital to articulate clearly the needs of children and families, to agree common eligibility criteria across services, to plan cohesive service improvement, and to aid the establishment of a sound research and evidence base for children's palliative care. It is anticipated that the discussions and debate currently under way through ACT and the International Children's Palliative Care Network will result in a consensus of terms to assist the future development of practice, service development, research and education.

Developing services

Much has been learnt from the development of children's palliative care services since the early 1980s. Many services, because of funding limitations, have developed in an ad hoc way that has resulted in inequity of provision (or at times a duplication of services), poor co-ordination between services, and stretched resources delivered by small teams of dedicated professionals (Craft and Killen 2007). Yet, at the same time, a worldwide consensus on the core elements of children's palliative care is emerging (see Figure 11.1), alongside a greater understanding of the need for partnership working to enable the full range of children's and family's needs to be met in an integrated, seamless way.

Transition to adult services

There are estimated to be between 6,000 and 10,000 young people living with a palliative care need in the UK (ACT 2007) and this number is set to increase as medical technology and therapies develop, and more young people survive into adulthood. Many young people are now reaching adulthood and finding that dedicated services to meet their needs do not exist to improve their experience of moving on to adult services. For many young people, their development into adulthood coincides with deteriorating health and greater dependence on carers. The differences between children's and adult services mean that there needs to be early planning for the transition and for preparatory work with the young person and his/her family to enable the shift to be made to a more young-person-centred,

- Flexible, integrated and co-ordinated services which recognize each child's and family's strengths and needs, enabling families to pursue ordinary lives and see their children achieve their full potential.

- Services delivered as a continuum of care from the time of diagnosis through death and bereavement.

- Timely and accurate communication and information between families and all services contributing to the child's care.

- Culturally sensitive services which also respond to emotional, social and spiritual needs.

- Interdisciplinary and interagency partnerships across health, social care, education and statutory and voluntary organizations.

- A choice of flexible short breaks.

- Appropriate and accessible funding arrangements.

- Access to a network of palliative care specialists.

- Planned, co-ordinated transition to appropriate adult services determined through the development of a multiagency plan centred on the wishes of the young person, acknowledging his/her right to plan proactively for the future (ACT 2007b).

- Planned emergency and end-of-life care to enable the child to die in his/her preferred place of care.

Figure 11.1 Core elements of children's palliative care

Sources: Adapted from (DH 2008, DHSSPS 2007, American Academy of Pediatrics (AAP) 2000 (reaffirmed 2007), Welsh Assembly Government 2006, Irish Hospice Association 2005, European Association of Palliative Care 2006, Australian Government Department of Health and Ageing (2004).

rather than family-centred, approach to care. The need for children's and adult services to work together is paramount if the young person and family are to experience a seamless transition.

Transition is not only of concern for service providers, but is also now a key government issue. The Department of Health (England) is initiating and developing a Transition Support Programme that will be rolled out across England. A number of resources have been developed to try to provide guidance on this issue, including the *Transition Care Pathway* (ACT 2007) and Transition: Moving On Well (DCFS and DH 2008).

=== **WEB LINKS** ===

Go to: www.transitioninfonetwork.org.uk and explore the work of the Transition Information Network, an alliance of organizations that have come together to improve the experience of young people with disabilities who are making the transition to adulthood.

Improving efficiency

Alongside these core components sits the need for cost-efficient service commissioning and delivery, and the need for service providers to develop effective partnerships with their local commissioning colleagues. As population demographics change, treatment options grow in range and cost and societal expectations expand, the government requirement to ensure the total health care benefits gained from money spent has never been more pressing. A central requisite of future children's palliative care services will be both to ensure and to provide evidence of their cost efficiency. This will not be a simple task, as it is difficult to quantify the benefits gained by promoting and protecting the wellbeing of families, or through utilizing alternative models of care. However, there is growing evidence to support the premise that community-based children's palliative care teams can deliver services valued by families and in a cost-effective manner (York Health Economics Consortium 2007). As we have seen, the number of children requiring a palliative approach to care comprises only a small percentage of the population, but palliative care services are expensive. It has been estimated that greater efficiency will be achieved through commissioning services for a population of at least one million people (York Health Economics Consortium 2007, DH 2008).

There are, therefore, likely to be considerable advantages in joint planning and commissioning arrangements across health trusts/primary care trusts and local authorities. This concept is currently being embraced across the UK, with the development of children's palliative care networks. The Welsh Assembly Government (2006) has indicated a commitment to commissioning local and specialist palliative care services on an all-Wales basis, and there is now a Scottish Children's and Young People's Palliative Care Network, which has developed a national vision for children's palliative care. Strategic health authorities across England are developing networks to bring together commissioners, professionals and services from the full range of disciplines and agencies involved. Such networks will aid the development of a 'sophisticated relationship' between statutory and voluntary services, thereby enabling services to augment local service provision and to deliver the best outcomes for children and families (DH 2008).

═══════════════════ **WEB LINKS** ═══════════════════

Find out about your regional or national children's palliative care network and get involved with their work by visiting the ACT website at: www.act.org.uk.

Improving data

A major issue for service commissioners, providers and service users is the lack of robust information on the number of children requiring palliative support, the services currently available, and whether these services are meeting individuals' needs. Such information is essential to influence policy and strategic development, to inform commissioning and enable integrated working, and to identify gaps and inequalities in service provision. A number of current databases, including local public health statistics, morbidity and mortality registers, Health for All Children databases and disabled children's registers hold components of this information, but bringing it together remains a challenge. In response, ACT and Children's Hospices UK are facilitating the implementation of a minimum data set for children's palliative care, and a service mapping tool to enable the collation of accurate information to inform local commissioning and quality assurance processes and facilitate national comparisons between regions.

================ **WEB LINKS** ================

Further updates on the roll-out and implementation of the minimum data set will be available through ACT and Children's Hospices UK. Available at: www.act.org.uk or www.childhospice.org.uk

Ensuring quality in children's palliative care

Quality in health and social care has many dimensions, and delivering quality services is not a passive process. Knowledge of effective care alone rarely leads to widespread improvement 'without a deliberate effort being made to change practice' (World Health Organization 2004: 22). Quality assurance processes need to be built into the fabric of every service and interlinking system through which collaborative care is delivered. Organizations are required by statute to monitor and improve the quality of health and personal social services provided to individuals, and a number of processes help to achieve this, such as the development of core standards. A range of useful standards have been developed through the National Service Framework for Children, Young People and Maternity Services (DH 2004), All Wales Standards for Palliative Care Services (2006) and the National Institute of Clinical Excellence Guidance on Children and Young People with Cancer (NICE 2005), for example. These standards may prove to be a useful tool to develop individual services, and to use as evidence of service performance by commissioning organizations.

Care pathways provide one approach to achieving co-ordinated care. Care pathways are standardized care plans that detail steps in patient care for specific illnesses, and list the expected treatments and progress for those patients (Campbell *et al.* 1998). Such a pathway has now been developed for children requiring palliative care (ACT 2004). This pathway is intended as a model to be adapted to meet local need. It incorporates five standards against which local services (or networks of services) can evaluate current provision, identifying areas of best practice as well as gaps that need to be addressed. ACT has further refined the standards into a comprehensive self-assessment tool to aid this process (available from ACT).

================ **WEB LINKS** ================

Consider using the self-assessment tool to evaluate your current service and to inform managers of the findings to aid future service development. Available at: www.act.org.uk

■ Benchmarks. There is a requirement for all nurses to ensure that care delivered is based on current evidence or best practice (Nursing and Midwifery Council 2008). Benchmarks provide a useful tool to assess current practice objectively and to implement steps for improvement. This process is further enhanced when undertaken simultaneously across a number of services, thereby increasing the opportunities for shared learning. Children's Hospices UK has an established benchmarking group which has assessed more than twenty distinct areas of practice.

CLINICAL FOCUS

Consider establishing a benchmarking group to share information and develop your service. You may find the benchmarks developed by Children's Hospices UK are useful aids. Contact Children's Hospices UK via their website for further advice, on www.childhospice.org.uk

Involving children and families

Service improvement does not sit only in the domain of professionals. Children and families themselves have a statutory right to contribute to the development and delivery of services. It is recognized that involving patients in decisions about health care at both personal and strategic levels is fundamentally important to the improvement of health and social care services, and leads to the provision of services that are more responsive to needs, to improved communication between organizations, patients and communities, and to greater ownership of services (NHS 2005). This is no less relevant in children's palliative care. Bodies responsible for assessing the performance of health care organizations, such as the Healthcare Commission in England and the Regulation and Quality Improvement Authority in Northern Ireland, seek evidence of engagement and involvement with service as part of the inspection process focusing on quality improvement. Such involvement can take may forms: seeking informal feedback, monitoring concerns and complaints, or employing user-satisfaction questionnaires and focus groups. However, the greatest benefits will be made through creating genuine, ongoing partnerships, where parents and professionals working together are acknowledged as each having a contribution to make to service planning and review, and are treated as equals (NHS 2005). Examples of such partnerships include the Children's and Young People Council at Alder Hey Children's Hospital, and the parent forum and young people's group ('Sixth Sense') established through the 'Wraparound' scheme. This aims to develop new and distinctive ways of multi-professional and multi-agency working to make a difference to the lives of children in the Southern Area of Northern Ireland.

KEY POINT

Achieving excellence in children's palliative care requires children and their families to be at the centre of service planning, delivery and evaluation.

Education*

The importance, contribution and value of a fit-for-purpose workforce is critical to ensuring high-quality care and support for life-limited children, young people and their families. As well as ensuring the necessary skills are developed within the existing workforce, it is important to consider succession planning to ensure future sustainability.

There is a need for a knowledge of children's palliative care at all levels of service, ranging from universal through to specialist services. A particular need is for the development of expertise in symptom control and end-of-life care that needs to be clinically driven, and developed as a collaboration between commissioners, service providers and the relevant Royal Colleges.

It is recommended that a collaborative approach is taken to meeting education and training needs along an education and training pathway that satisfies the requirements of all involved in the care of life-limited children and young people, from parents/carers to medical specialists. Such an approach would enable:

- national standards across the whole children's palliative care workforce;
- core standards for curriculum development (including standardized learning outcomes) across different groups and levels; and
- ways of acquiring Continuing Professional Development (CPD) points.

Taking the example of the stages of a care pathway that takes a child from recognition that his or her care is going to be palliative rather than curative, through living with the condition to the end-of-life stage, at each point the various levels of expertise and specialism are outlined in Figure 11.2.

It is essential that appropriately trained and skilled staff are available at each of the levels of service provision across the range of agencies, and in a variety of settings, throughout the care pathway.

All three levels of services need access to the whole range of tiers described in the Learning Cone model (see Figure 11.3).

The key aspects of this tiered approach to learning and development are that the whole workforce can:

- 'Hop on and off' the learning pathway to suit personal and professional needs.
- Enter the learning pathway at the relevant level.
- 'Bank' credits for learning.
- Study a range of accredited and non-accredited options at all levels.
- Benefit from a blended learning approaches.
- Take up opportunities for extensive workplace learning.

---

* Acknowledgements to Linda Maynard, Head of Education and Development at East Anglia's Children's Hospices, and to ACT and Children's Hospices UK for allowing us to use their developing Education and Training strategy in this section.

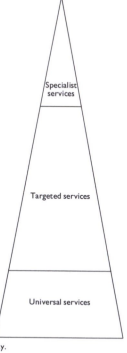

Diagnosis/recognition stage of care pathway*

Services should provide specialist investigations to enable accurate diagnosis or specialist services should be able to recognise when active treatment is no longer an option and refer appropriately to palliative care services. These are highly specialist services, involving the care of patients with more complex needs. They require specialist expertise.

Specialist services are analogous to secondary or tertiery health care services but may be provided in a range of settings including the child's home, school or other community setting, hospice or hospital. There is a major contribution at this level from disease-specific voluntary sector agencies such as CLIC Sargent; Debra; L.A. specialist children's teams, e.g. disability services; Hospice and other voluntary organisations and CCN services.

Services should provide appropriate investigations to enable accurate diagnosis and referral to specialist services if required. Services should also be able to provide emotional support to family members during this time.

Practical support to facilitate discharge home e,.g. transport; equipment provision. These services may include input from health care professionals with additional training and experience in palliative care (e.g. GPs with special interest), local authority specialist respite services, some aspects of provisions from children's hospice services and provision from other voluntary sector agencies such as the Jessie May Trust and Rainbow Trust; paediatric services (hospital/community); CCN services pathology services; psychological support; specialist Early Years Programmes; interpreters; specialist housing workers.

Services should enable a clear recognition and referral process to enable diagnosis and subsequent referral to required services. These services should be able to provide a palliative approach to their care, without referral to specialist palliative care units or personnel.

Primary Health Care Services including GP Services; Health Visiting; School Nursing; Opticians; Pharmacy; Midwifery Services; Newborn screening; Leisure and Play Services; Housing; Surestart; Early Years Programmes.

Specialist services

Targeted services

Universal services

* ACT Integrated Multi-agency care pathway.

Living with the condition

Services should contribute specialist information to multi-agency assessments and reviews and may provide a keyworker.

Specialist support e.g. supported short breaks as provided by children's hospice services and other voluntary sector agencies such at the Jessie May Trust and Rainbow Trust; Services may also include disease specific specialists; specialist children's teams e.g. disability services: specialised symptom management teams/ professionals.

Services should contribute to multi-abgency assessments and reviews and may provide a keyworker.

Services may include a paediatric service; pathology services; psychological support; specialist Early Years Programmes; interpreters; specilaist housing workers; 24 hour advice on management of pain and symptom management; therapy services; CCN services; specialist outreach services e.g. oncology; continuing care packages; CAMHS; Special Education Services; short breaks; specilaist housing; social care; hospice and other voluntary organisations.

Services should contibute to multi-agency assessments and reviews.

Services may include: Primary Health Care Services including GP Services; Health Visiting; School Nursing; Opticians; Pharmacy; Midwifery Services; New born screening; Leisure and Play Services; Housing; Surestart; Early Years Programmes.

Specialist services

Targeted services

Universal services

Figure 11.2 Three stages of an integrated multiagency care pathway

Source: Reproduced from ACT (2004), with the kind permission of ACT.

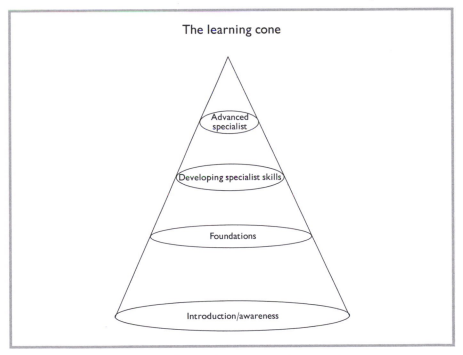

End of life care

Services should provide 24hr access to specialist care and advice as required by children, families and carers, including professional members of the care team.

Services should provide day-to-day care of the child and family and should have access to 24hr specialist advice through effective clinical networks.

Services should support the whole family emotionally and practically. Services to support the siblings of children and young people who are dying are an important part of supporting the whole family.

Specialist services

Targeted services

Universal services

Services may include specialist palliative care teams/professionals; disease specific/specialist palliative care: e.g. Neuro-disability Cystic Fibrosis and Muscula Dystrophy to enable effecive symptom management of severe, chronic pain and other distressin symptoms.

Services may include paediatric services; psychological support interpreters; therapy services' CCN services; Special Education Services; specialist housing; social care; hospice and other voluntary organisations; foster care.

Primary Health Care Services including GPO Services; Health Visiting; School Nursing; Opticians; Pharmacy; Midwifery Sservices; New born screening; Leisure and Play Services; Housing; Surestart; Early Years Programmes, Education services.

Figure 11.2   Continued

The learning cone

Advanced specialist

Developing specialist skills

Foundations

Introduction/awareness

Figure 11.3   The Learning Cone model

Source: ACT and Children's Hospices UK (2008). Reproduced with the kind permission of the ACT and Children's Hospices UK Education and Training Working Party, and Dr Linda Maynard, Head of Education and Development, East Anglia's Children's Hospices.

There are four key learning areas in the field of children's palliative care:

- communication skills;

- assessment skills;

- complex care, including symptom control; and

- role development.

This tiered approach to developing education and training builds on the notion that a wide range of learning approaches should be available. These will range ideally from attendance at one-day events and workshops to developing skills to become a consultant (nursing or medical) in the field of children's palliative care. An integrated approach to developing an education and training framework would enable the workforce to develop their competence levels and move through the skills escalator in a manner that better meets the needs of a total service pathway.

KEY POINT

The integrated care pathway can also help to define the core skills and competencies required across the interdisciplinary team as well as influencing the development of cohesive and comprehensive services for children's palliative care.

Research

In Chapter 1 of this book, lack of a substantive research base was highlighted. Throughout this text each chapter has drawn on the existing relevant research that can assist in care provision for children and families.

While the research base is increasing (ACT and RCPCH 2003), the development of a more robust research and evidence base is necessary, not only to refine our understanding and practice of children's palliative care but also to assist families (and practitioners supporting them) in making important decisions regarding the care or treatment of their children.

A number of difficulties have been identified when undertaking research in this field, including:

- The rarity of conditions.

- Ethical considerations of perceived benefits versus risks.

- Difficulties in identifying when some children are entering the palliative or end-of-life phases.

- The reliance on 'proxy' opinions from parents when children are unable to participate directly.

- Weak measurement tools.

- Methodological difficulties in establishing randomized control trials (Higginson 1999).

Internationally, a number of common topics have been proposed as priorities for research (American Academy of Pediatrics 2000, ACT and RCPCH 2003, Bosma *et al.* 2006). These priorities include:

- Incidence, prevalence, morbidity and mortality studies.

- Evaluation of therapeutic approaches to symptom management.

- Methods for improving communication and decision-making.

- Development of relevant outcome and validation measures including quality of life, particularly when death is expected in the foreseeable future (Institute of Medicine 2002).

- Evaluation of outcomes of integrating assessment and care co-ordination through the child's pathway.

- Cost–effectiveness analysis of various service delivery models.

- Bereavement care.

- Sibling support.

- Perinatal death.

- Educational needs analysis to develop a multiprofessional, skilled workforce.

Such research will require a multiprofessional approach across medicine, nursing, social work and other disciplines (ACT and RCPCH 2003). As the numbers of children involved are small, there is a growing call for organizations to collaborate to improve the collection of data (AAP 2000). The emergence of children's palliative care networks and the growing appointment of medical and nursing consultants for children's palliative care in the UK are expected to have a positive influence on a growing research base, as is the forthcoming appointment in the UK of a Chair in Palliative Care for Children and Young People. A further exciting development is the proposed establishment of an All Ireland Institute for Hospice and Palliative Care. A strategic objective of the proposed Institute is to become a leading international centre of expertise and information on education, research, policy and practice in palliative and end-of-life care. While the focus will remain on adult palliative care, the potential exists for researchers and practitioners to influence its research agenda to include children's palliative care.

The international network for children's palliative care

Children's palliative care is becoming a major international issue of concern, as it is becoming recognized that every child with a life-limiting or life-threatening condition should be able to access the best quality of life and care regardless of the country in which they live (International Children's Palliative Network 2007). The scale of the need for international recognition and development of children's palliative care is immense:

- Almost 40 per cent of admissions to hospice programmes in South Africa in 2005–6 were children and young people aged under 21 years.

- A national study in Germany indicated that the majority of children dying from cancer did not have access to comprehensive palliative care services at home (Friedrichsdorf *et al.* 2005).

- Access to pain-relieving medications is greatly impaired in resource-limited settings.

- A cultural denial of childhood death in some countries restricts the development of children's palliative care services (ICPCN 2007).

The international children's palliative care network has been established to facilitate dialogue between professionals and international organizations, to share information, raise awareness and to lobby governments to recognize and include children's palliative care on their strategic agendas.

WEB LINKS

Visit the ICPCN's website for further information on the global context of children's palliative care. Available at: www.icpcn.org

---

Conclusion

Since the late 1970s there has been considerable development and consolidation of children's palliative care. This has been driven by the energy and persistence of families and professionals, often working together to get their voice heard. Strategic direction has now been embedded in policy, placing the rights and needs of children, including children with life-limiting or life-threatening conditions, high on the political agenda (Welsh Assembly 2006, DHSSPS 2007, DH 2008). Full implementation of the recommendations contained within these reports will deliver the step change to improve the outcomes and experiences of all children requiring palliative care (DH 2008), yet much still remains to be done. Local commissioning arrangements encourage local authorities to determine their priorities and how services are configured and delivered. The development of local leadership, enhanced through collaborative working, ideally through a network approach, will be required to persuade and support commissioners and providers to deliver the changes children and families need.

It is through the development of individual practice, however, that so much can still be achieved to improve the care of life-limited children/young people and their families. We all need to reflect on the way that we work, communicate with each other and with families, and continue to develop partnerships across disciplines and agencies. We should all be mindful and informed about the challenging ethical issues that face us in children's palliative care, and ensure that the full range of support is in place, not only for the child but also for his or her parents, siblings and wider family. This care embraces the clinical and symptom control aspects of the child's care as well as the child and family's needs relating to a choice of flexible short breaks, and psychological, social and spiritual support. Everyone involved in children's palliative care will be working towards ensuring that all families receive timely support to help them to make end-of-life plans, and in providing a high quality of bereavement support for as long as it is needed.

Key resources

ACT (Association for Children's Palliative Care) (2004) *Framework for the Development of Multi-Agency Care Pathways for Life-limited Children.* Bristol: ACT.

DH (Department of Health) (2008) *Better Care: Better Lives: Improving Outcomes and Experiences for Children, Young People and Families Living with Life-limiting and Life-threatening Conditions.* London: Department of Health.

A selection of information and resources to assist in the improvement of services is available through the NHS Institute for Innovation and Improvement at: www.institute.nhs.uk The Improvement Leaders' Guides are particularly helpful booklets.

CHAPTER SUMMARY

- Children's palliative care is now recognized in its own right.

- The development of a strong policy base provides an opportunity to develop and deliver the agreed elements of a robust children's palliative care service.

- Confirming a common language for children's palliative care is essential, to articulate clearly the needs of children and families.

- A continual commitment to service improvement and efficiency is required.

- Delivery of quality in children's palliative care will rely on the education and development of a skilled and competent workforce that straddles the interdisciplinary interface and the establishment of a strong research base.

- The global context for children's palliative care will become increasingly relevant, providing both the opportunity to drive improvements in poorer countries and to participate in collaborative, international research to further increase the knowledge base.

References

ACT (Association for Children's Palliative Care) (2004) *Framework for the Development of Multi-Agency Care Pathways for Life-limited Children.* Bristol: ACT.

ACT (Association for Children's Palliative Care) (2007) *The Transition Care Pathway: A Framework for the Development of Integrated Care Pathways for Young People with Life-threatening and Life-limiting Conditions.* Bristol: ACT.

ACT (Association for Children's Palliative Care) and Children's Hospices UK (2008) A Practical Guide to Commissioning Children's Palliative Care, Education and Training: Planning and Developing an Effective and Responsive Workforce. A draft consultation document. Available at: www.act.org.uk/dmdocuments/A%20Commissioning%20Framework%20for%20Education%20and%20Training%20final%20draft%2008.doc

ACT and RCPCH (Association for Children with Life-Threatening or Terminal Conditions and their Families and Royal College of Paediatrics and Child Health (2003) *A Guide to the Development of Children's Palliative Care Services*, 2nd edn Bristol: ACT.

American Academy of Pediatrics (2000) Palliative care for children. *Pediatrics* **106**(2): 351–7.

Australian Government Department of Health and Ageing (2004) *The National Palliative Care Programme: Paediatric Palliative Care Service Model Review; Final Report.* Canberra: Australian Government Department of Health and Aging.

Bosma, H., Johnston, M. F., Cadell, S., Davies, B., Siden, H., Steele, R., Straatman, L. and Fleming, C. (2006) *Research in Pediatric Palliative Care: A Delphi Study.* Available at: www.pallpedsnet.ca/presentations.htm; accessed 10 April 2008.

Campbell, H., Hotchkiss, R., Bradshaw, N. and Porteous, M. (1998) Integrated care pathways. *British Medical Journal:* 133–7.

Craft A. and Killen S.(2007) *Palliative Care Services for Children and Young People in England: An Independent Review for the Secretary of State for Health.* London: Department of Health. Available at: www.dh.gov.uk/en/Publicationsandstatistics/Publications/PublicationsPolicyAndGuidance/DH_074459

DCFS and DH (Department for Children, Schools and Families, and Department of Health) (2008) *Transition: Moving on Well. A Good Practice Guide for Health Professionals and Their Partners on Transition Planning for Young People with Complex Health Needs or a Disability.* London: DCFS and DH.

DH (Department of Health) (2004) *National Service Framework for Children, Young People and Maternity Services: Executive Summary.* London: Department of Health.

DH (Department of Health) (2008) *Better Care: Better Lives: Improving Outcomes and Experiences for Children, Young People and Families Living with Life-limiting and Life-threatening Conditions.* London: Department of Health.

DHSSPS (Department of Health, Social Services and Public Safety) and University of Ulster (2007) *Complex Needs – The Nursing Response to Children and Young People with Complex Physical Healthcare Needs.* Belfast: DHSSPS.

European Association of Palliative Care (2006) IMPaCCT: standards for paediatric palliative care in Europe. *European Journal of Palliative Care* **14**(3): 2–7.

Friedrichsdorf, S. J., Menke, A., Brun, S., Wamsler, C. and Zernikow, B. (2005) Status quo of palliative care in pediatric oncology – a nationwide survey in Germany. *Journal of Pain and Symptom Management* **29**(2): 156–64.

Hewitt-Taylor, J. (2005) Caring for children with complex and continuing health care needs. *Nursing Standard* **19**(42): 41–7.

Higginson, I. (1999) Evidence based palliative care: there is some evidence – and there needs to be more. *British Medical Journal* **319**: 462–3.

Institute of Medicine (2001) *Crossing the Quality Chasm: A New Health System for the 21st Century.* Washington, DC: National Academy Press.

Institute of Medicine (2002) *When Children Die: Improving Palliative and End of Life Care for Children and Their Families.* Washington, DC: National Academies Press.

International Children's Palliative Care Network (2007) *The Need for Children's Palliative Care.* Available at: www.icpcn.org.uk; accessed 11 April 2008.

Irish Hospice Association/ Department of Health and Children (2005) *A Palliative Care Needs Assessment for Children.* Dublin: The Irish Hospice Foundation.

NHS Institute for Innovation and Improvement (2005) *Involving Patients and Carers: General Improvement Skills*. Nottingham: NHS.

NICE (National Institute for Clinical Excellence) (2005) *Improving Outcomes in Children and Young People with Cancer*. Available at: www.nice.org.uk

Nursing and Midwifery Council (2008) *The Code: Standards of Conduct, Performance and Ethics for Nurses and Midwives*. London: NMC.

Steele, R. (2000) Trajectory of certain death at an unknown time with degenerative life-threatening illness. *Cancer Journal of Nursing Research* **32**: 49–67.

UK Parliament (1989) *Children Act*. London: Stationery Office Stationery Office Ltd.

UK Parliament (1995) *Children (Northern Ireland) Order*. London: Stationery Office Ltd.

UK Parliament(1995) *Children (Scotland) Act*. London: Stationery Office Ltd.

Welsh Assembly Government (2006) *Children and Young People's Specialised Services Project: All Wales Standards for Palliative Care Services* (Consultation document). Cardiff: Welsh Assembly Government.

WHO (2004) *The Solid Facts: Palliative Care*. Copenhagen: World Health Organization.

York Health Economics Consortium (2007) *Independent Review of Palliative Care Services for Children and Young People: Economic Study*. York: University of York.

Index

adjuvant therapy, pain management   151
adult services, transition to   214–15
advance directives   81–2
after death   184–8
   see also bereavement care
age
   communication and   42
   competence and   72
   consent and   73
aids and equipment   115–16
alternative medicine   144
anniversaries   203
antibiotics for infection   165
anticipatory grief   193–4
anxiety   145
art   56
artificial nutrition and hydration   78
artificial ventilation   75
assent to treatment   73–4
assisted suicide   80–1
Association for Children with
   Life-threatening or Terminal
   Conditions and their Families (ACT)
   2, 6, 18, 40
   integrated care pathways   31
Association for Children's Palliative Care
   2, 6
Association of Children's Hospices UK   6
autonomy   68, 72

bad news, communication of   44–8
basic care concept   76
beneficence   68

benefits   *see* welfare benefits
bereavement care   192–3, 209
   accepting reality   201
   adjusting to new reality   202
   anticipatory grief   193–4
   developing self-awareness   196–8
   experiencing pain or emotional aspects of
      the loss   201–2
   listening to bereaved families   198–200
   looking after ourselves   207–8
   process of grieving   200
   siblings   205–7
   ways of remembering   202–5
   working with bereaved families   195–6
bleeding   162–3
boundaries   204

cancer   5, 9, 46
cardiopulmonary resuscitation   79–80
   do-not-resuscitate (DNR) status   43, 165
chaplain   22, 138, 144, 182
children
   autonomy   68, 72
   competence   72–3
   consent issues   67, 73–4
   growth and development   12
   palliative care for   *see* palliative care for
      children
   rights of   7, 65–7, 213
   spiritual needs   *see* spiritual needs of
      children and families
   support for   *see* supporting children and
      families

Children Act 1989   66
Children Act 2004   66
Children's Workforce Network   19
communication   38, 58
  barriers to   40–2
  breaking bad news   44–8
  challenges within children's palliative care
    43
  communicating with children about death
    50, 52–7
  context in children's palliative care   39–40
  decision-making and   70
  definitions   39
  ethical issues   74–5
  negotiating tensions and conflict   57–8
  sharing information   48–52
community-based palliative care   10, 173
community children's nurses   10, 22, 27, 29,
    40–1, 42, 116, 131, 162
competence   72–3
complementary medicine   144
confidentiality   114
conflict
  communication and   57–8
  ethical issues and   68, 70
  in teamwork   26
consent issues   67, 73–4
  parental consent   74
constipation   156–9
co-ordination schemes   28
  integrated care pathways   31
  keyworking   28–30
  'Team Around the Child'   30–1
cough   159
counselling   113
culture
  bereavement and   197
  end-of-life care and   181–2
  reflection and   139

data, improving   216–17
death
  achieving a 'good death'   183–4
  after death   184–8
  communicating with children about   50,
    52–7
  end-of-life decisions   75–6
  inability to accept   42
  stages of dying   47, 53
  see also bereavement care
decision-making   67, 69–72
  end-of-life care   179–81
  see also end-of-life decisions
denial   42, 57–8
depression   145

diamorphine   151
dietician   10, 22, 162
diarrhoea   159
disability   213
  Disability Living Allowance (DLA)
    114–15
  UN Convention on the Rights of Persons
    with Disabilities   66, 67
diversity, in teams   21
doctors   9, 22, 26, 27, 45, 46, 131, 143, 146,
    162, 185, 187
Dominica, Frances   6
do-not-resuscitate (DNR) status   43, 165
drawing   56
drugs   *see* pharmacological management
dyspnoea   159–61

Ecomap   120–2
education
  future directions for palliative care and
    219–22
  inter-professional education (IPE)   32
efficiency   216
emotions   47, 48, 109
  emotional support   112–14
  experiencing pain or emotional aspects of
    the loss   201–2
end-of-life care   172, 188
  decision-making   179–81
  history and policy context   172–5
  initial assessment of end-of-life care needs
    177–8
  pain management   178–9
  pathways   176–7
  quality of life   181
  recognition of end-of-life stage   177
  seizures during   147
  spiritual, religious and cultural issues
    181–2
  symptom management   163–4, 178–9
  time of death   183–4
end-of-life decisions   75–6, 164
  antibiotics for infection   165
  'do-not-resuscitate' order   43, 165
  drug regime   164
  feeding   164–5
epilepsy   145–6
equipment   115–16
ethical issues   64, 83
  advance directives   81–2
  approaches to ethics   68–9
  artificial nutrition and hydration   78
  assisted suicide   80–1
  autonomy   68, 72
  cardiopulmonary resuscitation   79–80

competence   72–3
consent   67, 73–4; parental consent   74
context of ethics   67–8
decision-making   67, 69–72; end-of-life
    decisions   75–6
euthanasia   80
genetic testing   82–3
legal aspects   65
long–term ventilation   75
organ donation and transplantation   82
parental responsibility   65
reflection and   139
rights of the child   65–7
sanctity of life   80
truth telling   74–5
withdrawing and withholding treatment
    76–7
euthanasia   80

families   *see* parents and families
Family Law Reform Act   1969   66
feeding *see* nutrition, artificial
financial support   114
    direct payments   115
    Disability Living Allowance (DLA)
    114–15
funeral director   186, 187
funerals   186, 187
future directions for palliative care   213–14,
    224–5
    developing services   214
    education   219–22
    ensuring quality   217–18
    improving data   216–17
    improving efficiency   216
    international networks   223–4
    involving children and families   218
    refining the language   214
    research   222–3
    transition to adult services   214–15

gastro-oesophageal reflux (GER)   153–6
gender, emotion and   47, 109
genetic illnesses   12
    genetic testing   82–3
grandparents   122
grief   196, 204
    anticipatory   193–4
    process of grieving   200
groupthink   26

haemorrhaging   162–3
health visitor   131
Helen House (Oxford)   6

historical development of palliative care for
    children   5–7
home adaptations   116
home care   172–4
hospice nurse   22, 27, 51, 131
hospices   3
    after death care   188
    children's hospices   6, 7, 10, 174–5
    development of palliative care and   1,
    5–6
    play specialists   9, 22, 45, 50, 51, 52, 56,
    131, 144
hospitals
    children's deaths in   10
    end-of-life care in   175, 183
hydration, artificial   78

information, communication of
    see communication
informed consent   73
integrated approach to palliative care   11
integrated care pathways   31
Integrated Qualifications Network   19
interdisciplinary teams   13–14, 18, 34
    benefits of team-working   23–4
    blurring and crossing boundaries   27–8
    care-co-ordination schemes   28;
        integrated care pathways   31;
        keyworking   28–30; 'Team Around
        the Child'   30–1
    children's palliative care team   22;
        enhancing performance   32–4;
        leadership   25–6; nature and
        dynamics   24–5; size of team   25
    conflict in teamwork   26
    health care team   21
    meaning of 'team'   20–1
    parents as members of team   23
    policy context   19
    reflecting and   130
    role ambiguity   27
    stages of team development   24
international networks for children's
    palliative care   4, 7, 40, 223–4
Internet   49
inter-professional education (IPE)   32

justice   68

Kennedy Report   19
key worker concept   28–30

Laming Report   19
leadership in children's palliative care team
    25–6

legal issues
  consent 73
  ethics and 65
withdrawing and withholding treatment
  76–7
life
  life-prolonging treatment concept 76
  sanctity of 80
listening to bereaved families 198–200
living wills (advance directives) 81–2
long-term ventilation 75

Macmillan nurse 22, 27, 51, 131
Mental Capacity Act 2005 66, 72
mental problems 144–5
'miracle cures' 49
mobility allowances 117
models of palliative care 9–11
money   *see* financial support
moral issues   *see* ethical issues
morphine 150
mortuaries 186
multidisciplinary teams   *see* interdisciplinary
  teams
muscle spasm 152
music therapy 103

National Children's Bureau 67
National Service Frameworks 19, 66
nausea and vomiting 152–3
non-maleficence 68
nurse 9, 22, 27, 45, 46, 83, 113, 119, 123,
  131, 185
nutrition, artificial 78
  end-of-life decisions and 164–5

occupational therapist 10, 22, 116, 131, 162
organ donation and transplantation 82

pain management 147–8
  adjuvant therapy 151
  end-of-life care 178–9
  experiencing pain or emotional aspects of
    the loss 201–2
  managing children's pain 148–50
  muscle spasm 152
  spiritual pain 151–2
  using diamorphine 151
  using morphine 150
palliative care for children 1–2, 13–14
  challenges 13
  classification of children requiring 3–4
  definitions and categories 2–4
  differences from adult care 11–13
  historical development 5–7

models 9–11
  prevalence of children requiring 4–5,
    12–13
  principles and philosophy 8–9
  see also individual topics
palliative care nurses 123–4
parents and families
  after death of child 186
  bereavement   *see* bereavement care
  communication with   *see* communication
  end-of-life care and 183–4
  end-of-life care decision-making 179–81
  future directions for palliative care and
    218
  involvement in palliative care 11–12
  parental consent 74
  parental responsibility 65
  parents as members of interdisciplinary
    teams 23
  philosophy of palliative care and 8–9
  spiritual needs   *see* spiritual needs of
    children and families
  support for   *see* supporting children and
    families
person-centred counselling 113
pet therapy 103
pharmacist 162
pharmacological management 143
  end-of-life decisions and 164
  seizures 146
philosophy of palliative care 8–9
physiotherapist 10, 22, 116, 131, 162
play 50–1, 56, 97
play specialist 9, 22, 45, 50, 51, 52, 56, 131,
  144
postmortem examinations 186
practical support 115–17
principles of palliative care 8–9
psychiatrist 145
psychological problems 144–5
psychologist 9, 145
psychosocial support 108–10

quality of children's palliative care 217–18
quality of life 181

Redfern Report 82
reflection 128–9, 139
  cultural/spiritual/ethical issues 139
  model for use in children's palliative care
    130–1; first (deductive) phase
    132–3; post-reflection phase 135–7;
    preliminary phase 131–2; second
    phase 133–4; third (inductive) phase
    134–5

reasons for   129–30
socio-political constraints   138–9
refusal of treatment   76–7
religion   91–2
    end-of-life care and   181–2
remembering   202–5
research
    future directions for palliative care   222–3
    Internet and other sources   49
respiration, excessive respiratory secretions
    161–2
respite   117–19
resuscitation   79–80
    do-not-resuscitate (DNR) status   43, 165
rights of the child   65–7
    UN Convention   7, 65, 66, 213
role ambiguity   27
Royal College of Paediatrics and Child
    Health (RCPCH)   2, 80

salivation, excessive   161–2
sanctity of life   80
Save the Children   67
schoolteachers   10, 22, 56, 113, 121, 131, 144,
    162, 177
seizures   145–7
    during end-of-life care   147
    persistent   146
self-awareness   196–8
siblings
    bereavement care and   205–7
    support from   119–22
situated ethics   69
social security   see welfare benefits
social workers   9, 22, 26, 27, 45, 113, 114,
    123, 131, 177
speech and language therapist   10, 22, 161
spiritual needs of children and families   88,
    104
    challenges of palliative care   102–3
    defining spirituality   89–91
    drivers for spiritual care   89
    end-of-life care and   181–2
    expression of   97, 98–100
    imperative questions   91
    limitations to provision of   103–4
    models representing spiritual dimension
        93
    reflection and   139
    religion and spirituality   91–2
    spiritual assessment   94–7
    spiritual care   97, 100–2
    spiritual pain   151–2
story-telling   50, 103
suicide assisted   80–1

supporting children and families   107–8,
    124
    assessment   110–11
    emotional support   112–14
    financial support   114; direct payments
        115; Disability Living Allowance
        (DLA)   114–15
    grandparents   122
    practical support   115–17
    psychosocial support   108–10
    respite   117–19
    sibling support   119–22
    types of support   112
symptom management   142–3, 165–6
    bleeding   162–3
    constipation   156–9
    cough   159
    diarrhoea   159
    dyspnoea   159–61
    end-of-life care   163–4, 178–9
    end-of-life decisions and   164; antibiotics
        for infection   165; drug
        regime   164; feeding   164–5; need
        for written 'do-not-resuscitate'
        order   165
    excessive salivary/repiratory secretions
        161–2
    gastro-oesophageal reflux (GER)   153–6
    general approach   143–4
    nausea and vomiting   152–3
    pain   147–8; adjuvant therapy   151;
        end-of-life care   178–9; managing
        children's pain   148–50; muscle
        spasm   152; spiritual pain   151–2;
        using diamorphine   151; using
        morphine   150
    psychological problems   144–5
    seizures   145–7

'Team Around the Child' approach   30–1
teamwork   see interdisciplinary teams
technology
    artificial nutrition and hydration
        see nutrition, artificial
    long-term ventilation   75
teenagers
    palliative care for   9
    transition to adult services   214–15
therapy   see treatment and therapy
transition to adult services   214–15
transplantation   82
transport   117
treatment and therapy
    artificial nutrition and hydration   78
    basic care concept   76

treatment and therapy (*continued*)
  consent issues 67, 73–4; parental consent 74
  life-prolonging treatment concept 76
  music therapy 103
  palliative *see* palliative care for children
  pet therapy 103
  withdrawing and withholding 76–7; living wills (advance directives) 76–7
  see also symptom management
truth telling 74–5

United Nations
  Convention on the Rights of Persons with Disabilities 66, 67
  Convention on the Rights of the Child (1989) 7, 65, 66, 213

ventilation 75
vomiting 152–3

welfare benefits
  direct payments 115
  Disability Living Allowance (DLA) 114–15
  mobility allowances 117
withdrawing and withholding treatment 76–7
living wills (advance directives) 76–7